M000313390

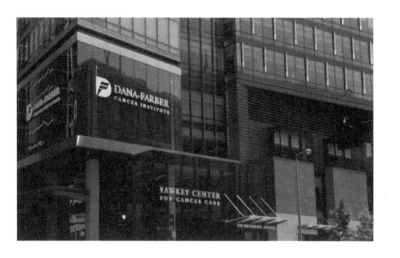

"BAD LUCK":

An Inspirational Journey in the Battle
Against Pancreatic Cancer

Written by
Michael J Florio

Table of Contents

INTRODUCTION

This story is about my journey and battle with pancreatic cancer. It is not intended to provide you with specific information about cancer itself. Anything contained within that is not specific to my journey was obtained by simply looking things up on-line, and so may be only somewhat accurate.

The National Cancer Institute defines cancer as a disease in which some of the body's cells grow uncontrollably and spread to other parts of the body. These cells may form tumors, larges lumps of tissue, which may be either cancerous or non-cancerous/benign. Cancerous tumors, also known as malignant tumors, may produce cells that can travel to other areas of the body to form new tumors in a process called metastasis. Metastatic cancer has the same name and the same type of cancer cells as the original cancer. For example, breast cancer that metastasizes in the lungs is referred to as metastatic breast cancer and not lung cancer. Most people that die of cancer, die from metastatic disease.

Although many cancers form solid tumors, cancers of the blood, such as leukemias, generally do not. Cancer cells do not behave the way normal cells do. Usually, when a cell divides, there is usually, at some point, a signal that tells the cell to stop replicating; with cancerous cells, that signal is lost, and the cells continue to divide. These cells may also spread to other areas of the body, preventing normal organ function. It is like an icemaker in your freezer that does not stop making ice when it is supposed to. If you can catch it before it spills out of the tray, then it is easily cleaned up. If, however, the ice overflows and falls out, it can move to all areas of the freezer, making it more difficult to remove.

Cancer is a genetic disease that is caused by changes to our genes that control the way cell's function, especially how cells grow and divide. These changes can occur due to damage to DNA caused by harmful substances in the environment or inherited traits from our parents. Normally our body eliminates cells with damaged DNA before they turn cancerous. However, as we age, our body's ability to do so diminishes. Hence, you are at a greater risk of developing cancer the older you become.

There are more than 100 different types of cancer. Types of cancer are usually named for the organs or tissues where the cancers form. For example, pancreatic cancer originates in the pancreas, while liver cancer starts in the liver. Cancers may also be described by the type of cell from which they are formed. For example, squamous cell or epithelial cell.

Carcinomas, formed by epithelial cells, are the most common type of cancer. Adenocarcinomas, like the type of cancer that I was diagnosed with, form in epithelial cells that produce fluids or mucus and are known as glandular tissues. Most cancers of the breast, colon, prostate, and pancreas are adenocarcinomas.

Basil cell carcinoma is a cancer that forms in the epidermis, the outer layer of the skin, while squamous cell carcinoma forms in squamous cells, epithelial cells that lie just beneath the epidermis. These cells are also found in many other organs, including the stomach, intestines, lungs, bladder, and kidneys. Transitional cell carcinoma also forms in epithelial tissues that line the bladder, ureters, and kidneys.

Sarcomas are cancers that form in bone and soft tissues, including muscle, fat, blood vessels, lymph vessels, tendons, and ligaments. Common types of sarcomas include leiomyosarcoma, Kaposi sarcoma, malignant fibrous histiocytoma, liposarcoma, and dermatofibrosarcoma protuberans.

Leukemias are cancers that begin in the bone marrow. They form when large numbers of abnormal white blood cells accumulate in the blood and bone marrow, displacing normal blood cells and preventing them from functioning properly. Because of this, it is harder for the body to get oxygen to the tissues, control bleeding and fight infections.

Lymphomas are cancers that begin in disease-fighting white blood cells known as lymphocytes. These cells may be classified as either T cells or B cells. In lymphoma, abnormal lymphocytes build up in lymph nodes and lymph vessels, as well as in other organs. There are two main types of lymphoma: Hodgkin lymphoma and non-Hodgkin lymphoma.

Multiple myeloma, also known as plasma cell myeloma or Kahler disease, is a disease that begins in a type of immune cell called a plasma cell. Myeloma cells build up in the bone marrow and form tumors in the bones themselves.

Melanomas are cancers of specialized cells called melanocytes, which produce melanin, a pigment that gives skin its color. Most melanomas form in the skin, but some can also form in other pigmented tissues, such as the eye.

Brain and spinal cord tumors derive their name based on the type of cell in which they are formed as well as where the tumor first formed in the central nervous system. These tumors, like others, may be benign (non-cancerous) or malignant (cancerous).

Germ cell tumors form in cells that produce sperm or eggs. These tumors can also occur almost anywhere in the body and can be either benign or malignant.

Neuroendocrine tumors develop from cells that release hormones into the blood. These tumors may cause an organ to make higher than-normal amounts of hormones. These tumors may also be benign or malignant. One type of neuroendocrine tumor is called a carcinoid tumor. These slow-growing tumors are usually found in the gastrointestinal system, usually the rectum and small intestine. Carcinoid tumors may spread to the liver or other sites in the body.

Information reference by: National Cancer Institute (gov)
https://www.cancer.gov>about-cancer>understanding

BAD LUCK

Bad luck. That's what I was told. It was just bad luck. Although so simple and without much meaning, it was an answer that I could understand. When we think about life, where we are, and what we are, is it all just luck or perhaps fate? Is our life predetermined? It is said that our life is about choices, but do we really decide? Why is it that we do the things that we do and make the choices we make? What causes one sibling to move halfway around the world and away from the home they grew up in while the other moves next door? What is the driving force that causes us to do things? Each day we are faced with a myriad of factors that influence and determine our destiny. Are these factors random, or do they follow some logical order? A simple, unexpected phone call can alter your entire life in the same way as a birth of a child, the death of a loved one, or the diagnosis of a certain medical condition. We have all experienced these things. Life can change in an instant; for better or for worse.

THE BEGINNING

My life story, for the most part, is like everyone else's. You could say that some are more fortunate than others, but collectively and in the end, we are similar in the trials and tribulations we all face. I was born and would become the only child of a hardworking and "traditional" family. Mom took care of the inside of the house and had dinner on the table every night, while Dad took care of everything on the outside, including all carpentry, plumbing, electrical and auto repair. You can say he was a "jack of all trades." My home was filled with love, security, and comfort. We lacked for nothing. What we could not afford to buy, my dad simply made or repaired.

Growing up across the street from the water, more specifically Clarks Cove, in the south end of the City of New Bedford, the birth place of Herman Melville's "Moby Dick," it wasn't surprising that at some point, I would want to have a boat of my own; and so, when I was just about entering my teenage years, my dad built a row boat in the basement of our home. He had never taken on such a task but was confident he could get it done. When the boat was just about near completion, my dad looked at it and said, "shit." He didn't really use cuss words, so I was kind of surprised he said this. I just looked at him with a questioning look, and he said, "I am not sure we are going to be able to get it out of the basement." Well, we did, and my dad was then tasked with building a hand trailer so the boat could be towed across the street and launched. I spent countless hours rowing and using it to swim off of. I was truly blessed to grow up in the kind of household I did.

I have always been physically active and still, to this day, enjoy working out and playing sports. I am very health conscious. I never smoked or took drugs, and I don't consume any alcohol. Even at my wedding, I had non-alcoholic champagne. I don't drink coffee, eat donuts or visit fast food restaurants such as McDonalds or Burger King. Although I do eat meat, mostly chicken or fish, the majority of my diet is plant-based. I have regular physical exams and visit the dentist every six months. I am not overweight and take no medications.

In 2018 after spending 34 years teaching in the New Bedford School System, I retired from teaching but continued working as a paramedic. In 1982, I became certified as an EMT and then as a paramedic in 2001. Even while teaching, I continued to work in the field of Emergency Medical Services. I have been working in an ambulance since I was 14, initially on an animal ambulance with the New Bedford Animal Rescue League. It has been an honor and privilege to have been able to help so many for a considerably long period of time, and I have been fortunate to have remained healthy enough to do so.

Without any real sense of direction as to what I would do after I retired from teaching, I just thought I would continue to work in the field of emergency medicine until I became too old to do so any longer. Then in 2019, the pandemic struck. At first, it was business as usual, but then things started to change as people around the world became sick and started dying. The policies at my worksites started to change, and I began to wear masks and gowns and completed self-health questionnaires and temperature checks before beginning my shift. I Wiped down the entire inside of the ambulance after every call.

Removed my work clothing in the basement of my home and washed them separately from other clothes. Life itself began to change. People kept their distance from others. One-way lines were set up in stores, and certain items began to disappear from shelves. Limits were placed on how much of a particular product you could buy at one time. Stickers were placed on the floor telling people were to stand at the checkout line so that they remained six feet from the next person. People began to work from home, and schools were closed. There was fear of contracting a potentially deadly illness, and yet here I was still, at nearly age 60, myself in a more at-risk group, going into people's homes, even in homes of people with known Covid, in order to provide emergency medical care.

Around that same time, I was still going to the YMCA every morning, where I would swim and take part in a yoga class. At one point, we had a substitute yoga instructor, and let's just say she would definitely help increase the male enrolment numbers. To me, one of the things that stood out when looking at her was her washboard abs. She had an incredibly strong core and did sit-ups effortlessly. I took this as a challenge, and so I also began to spend more time doing abdominal and core workouts. I had also been plagued with what I would call older person joint pain, and so against my better judgment, I went on-line and bought a product called Flexify, which came in a kind of orange color pill form. I also started taking Ibuprofen. I felt that the combination of the two would help with any inflammation I was having.

Here I was, relatively strong and healthy, the only medications now being Flexify and Ibuprofen, which I was taking on my own accord, and working around 40 hours/week. Things seemed to be going okay. On March 23, 2020, I was working on an ambulance and brought a patient to Charlton Memorial Hospital in Fall River, where one of my daughters was a nurse and where she just happened to be working at that time. After I dropped off my patient, my daughter kind of took me aside and said to me, "What are you doing? Mom is immunocompromised, and you are retired. You don't have to be working now during the pandemic." (For years, my wife has been dealing with chronic pancreatitis and other auto immune disorders, which have sometimes left her hospitalized for months.) Now, when your parents or significant other give you hell, you just kind of shrug your shoulders, but when your kids do, it is a completely different story, so on March 23, 2020, I stopped working; two weeks later, I started to get sick.

It started as abdominal discomfort, which I attributed to all the abdominal and core workouts I was doing. I also thought that perhaps the Ibuprofen and Flexify that I was taking might have upset my liver, which could also be contributing to my abdominal discomfort. It wasn't really pain, and on a scale of 1 – 10, I would have given it perhaps a 2 due to it constantly being there. At one point, over a weekend, I made an appointment to see my doctor but then canceled it because, for a brief moment, the abdominal discomfort seemed to disappear. Shortly thereafter, my urine started to turn a sort of orange color, which I attributed to the Flexify, but then my stool began to turn a sort of clay-like color. Although disgusting, it is important to note and be aware of the things that come out of you, pee and poop, for they can help determine your health. Any changes in odor, color, consistency, blood, pus, or mucus could be signs that you should be aware of and perhaps indicate the need to seek medical attention. I sort medical attention after I started losing weight. Before taking a shower and while admiring myself in a mirror, ouch, I noticed that I looked thinner, so I got off the bathroom scale and started to weigh myself each morning. What I discovered was that, despite eating regularly, I was losing a pound every day. My starting weight was 167 pounds, and when I got down to 159, I got scared, I don't mean worried or concerned, I mean, I was actually scared, and so I called my doctor. On April 8, 2020, I saw my general practitioner. I explained to him all of my signs and symptoms and told him I was taking Flexify and Ibuprofen. I also mentioned all of the abdominal workouts I was doing. When it comes to my health, I do not keep any secrets from any of my health care providers. I don't know why anyone would not tell the truth to those taking care of you. If you are going to be dishonest with them, don't bother seeking their assistance. People are afraid of being embarrassed, but embarrassment is a condition or feeling that you place on yourself. Truthfully, no one else cares, especially those providing medical assistance. As I sat across from my doctor, he looked at me and said, "So, in the middle of Covid, you have come here and presented a challenge to me, don't worry. We will figure it out." He sent me for blood work and an ultrasound of my bladder. I returned home, and around 4 o'clock in the afternoon, I received a call from my doctor's office. I was told that my ultrasound was normal. Five minutes later, my doctor's office called again and said that my blood work revealed elevated liver enzymes and that I was scheduled for another ultrasound the following day. I hung up the phone and thought to myself, I guess I was right. The Flexify and Ibuprofen have upset my liver.

THE DIAGNOSIS

On April 9, 2020, I found myself back at Hawthorn Medical in Dartmouth, Massachusetts, having another ultrasound. It seemed like I was lying on the ultrasound bed for a long time, perhaps half an hour, as a gel was placed all over my abdomen, and various images were being taken. Sort of abruptly, the technician stopped and said that she would be right back. I thought she had said that she was going to take more images of my vasculature, so I continued to lie on the bed. Again, it seemed like I was just lying there for quite a while, and the gel that she had placed on me dried up. My shirt was off, and I started to become cold, so I sat up, wiped myself off with a towel that had been lying around, and put my shirt back on. Suddenly, she came back in and said that my doctor would see me now. I said to myself, "I guess I am done. I thought she said she had more images to take." Initially, I was surprised that my doctor could see me right away. Then I thought that he must be available because no one was around. We were, after all, in the grip of a pandemic. I believed that he was going to say that nothing was found on the ultrasound and that he would continue to monitor my elevated liver enzymes. Then it occurred to me that perhaps something was found and that something may not be too good, but I thought, whatever, let me go see what he has to say. I was led back into an examination room. It did not take long before he walked in. He wasted no time in telling me that there was a 4 cm mass in the head of my pancreas and that I had cancer, and that he was sorry. He also said that in a little over 4 hours, he had me scheduled for an MRI. I asked him if I could have something to eat, and he said that I had 15 minutes to do so. I thought to myself, it is a good thing I brought some snacks with me. I don't even know why I thought about eating. I guess maybe because it was something I still had control over. When a doctor tells you that you have cancer, do you even hear anything else that is said after that? Even now, as I write these words, it is still very difficult to think about. It was around 9:45 a.m. when I was told. My MRI was scheduled for 2 p.m. 15 minutes to eat. I went to my car and ate the snacks I had brought with me. Truthfully, I don't remember what happened after that. I just don't know. I am assuming that I went home and told my wife, but I really can't remember. All I know is that at 2 p.m. I had an MRI which confirmed a 3.8 cm mass in the head of my pancreas. I think I just went home and sat on the couch for the rest of the night. Again, I don't remember much of that evening. I remember my wife letting my two daughters know of my diagnosis, and my daughter Mikayla, the one who gave me hell for working during Covid, saying, "wait, dad has pancreatic cancer?"

As stated before, my wife has suffered for years from chronic pancreatitis. I have always been healthy, so I think it came as more of a shock and surprise that I would be the one to develop this disease. Yet, here I was, trying to make sense of what I had just been told. My wife once said that if someone were to develop cancer, pancreatic was not the one to get. It is painful to go through, and the survival rate is poor. In fact, if you do a Google search, you will find that the 5-year survival rate is only 10%, and the 10-year survival rate is only 4%. Even if you take into account the strides made in recent years to combat this deadly disease and you doubled your chances of survival, the numbers are still pretty grim. The evening was spent on the couch, a place where I would end up spending a lot of time. I don't remember what I did, but probably nothing. I don't remember when I went to bed, but I do remember lying there and shaking. I couldn't believe that this was happening to me. I finally had to call out to my wife and tell her to come to bed with me. Her presence brought me comfort, and I was eventually able to fall asleep. The following day I canceled my YMCA membership and began to organize some of the things that I do around that house so that my wife would be able to understand what to do in case I was no longer capable of carrying out those tasks. Assuming that my hair was going to fall out after I began my treatment, I wondered what I would look like being bald and felt that it might be better to shave my head before my hair began to fall out. I went on Amazon to look for hair clippers, but my wife felt that it was best that I wait and see what happens after I begin my treatment. She said that it could be possible that I would not lose my hair. Many times, I also thought of calling the funeral parlor to make my arrangements but never could bring myself to do so. I don't recall what I did over the following days, for it all seems like a blur. I do remember that my wife posted my condition on Facebook and received nearly 800 responses. I had never been on Facebook before, and she recommended that I set up my own account. Through Facebook, I kept people informed about my entire journey. I also remember being prescribed Xanax to help me relax, but I did not start taking it until after I began chemo. I wish I had been given it the day of my diagnosis; I think it would have been very beneficial during that first night.

I don't exactly know when, but it was only a few days following my diagnosis that I began to turn yellow. I actually started to notice it in my chest first and then in the sclera of my eyes. Shortly thereafter, I was scheduled for an ERCP. Due to Covid restrictions, no visitors/family were ever allowed to accompany me to any of my procedures, and so everything I did, all of my surgeries, chemo, and radiation, would be done alone. I would be dropped off at the front door and then picked up when I was ready to come home. Sometimes it is kind of strange as to the things you remember, but just before going in for my ERCP, I went to the bathroom and looked to see how much toilet paper there was. My friend Joe had asked me if I could steal some for him. Because of Covid, it seems like, for some reason, there was a run-on toilet paper. I never understood why, but I guess Joe was having a difficult time finding some. I know that he was just joking, but as I think about it, maybe not.

During the ERCP, I stent was placed in my bile duct, and a biopsy was done on my tumor. The biopsy revealed that the tumor was an adenocarcinoma. A quick Google search will tell you that adenocarcinoma is the most common type of pancreatic cancer, and in general, the survival rate is very poor; this is because it is often detected in its later stages of development when it has already spread to other organs. Although I am a firm believer that one should be a strong advocate for one's own health and that you should learn as much as you can about your medical condition, it is important that you seek and listens to a doctor who specializes in your illness.

My ERCP was done on an out-patient basis, as I believe most are. I was sent home with the pain killer Vicodin as I am allergic to Percocet. Actually, I am not allergic to it. It just makes me nauseated. While at home, I suffered from severe abdominal pain and took Vicodin every 8 hours as directed. Although my jaundice was beginning to clear, I was miserable and quickly running out of pain medication. Because of this, I called my doctor, who had given me his personal number, and he told me that I should not still be having abdominal pain. He suggested that I go to Urgent Care. It was Friday, and Urgent Care would be closed during the weekend, which meant that if I needed medical attention, I would have to go to an emergency room, which he was concerned would be full of people with Covid. As I hung up the phone, I was a little upset with him. This was the first time that I actually disagreed with what a doctor told me. What was Urgent Care going to do for me? I felt that all I needed was pain meds. Anyway, I did what he instructed me to do and had my wife take me to Urgent Care. Again because of Covid restrictions, she was not able to go inside Urgent Care and was forced to wait in her car. I believe my doctor had notified them that I would be coming and had given them my medical history. I was examined, and an X-ray was taken. My doctor actually called me while I was there to discuss the result of the X-ray. He said that everything looked fine. The doctor at Urgent Care said that I was dehydrated, something I should have recognized myself due to the white coloration of my tongue. I was told to drink more fluids and was basically sent on my way. The odd thing is that I actually felt better. My abdominal pain was just about gone, and I did not need to take any more pain meds. To this day, I am not sure why that happened. Maybe by moving around, I unblocked something that had been blocked and caused pain; I don't know. I also had a better understanding of what to do in order to stay hydrated. It has been said that you should drink 8 glasses of water or other fluids each day. If each glass contains 8 ounces of fluid, then that would mean that you should be drinking 64 ounces a day. My Nalgene bottles have a capacity of 32 ounces, and therefore two bottles would be 64 ounces, just the amount recommended to remain adequately hydrated; and so, each morning, I would fill 2 bottles with water and drink them throughout the day. This all seemed to work for me because I started to feel better.

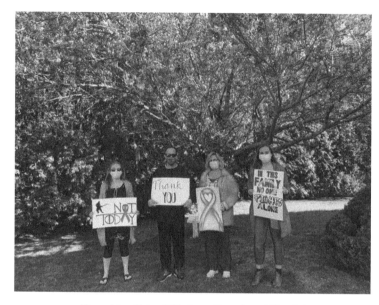

(Daughter Kate, Wife Ann, Daughter Mikayla)

TREATMENT BEGINS

The question now was, where do I go to seek treatment for my cancer? It was obvious that I would be going to a hospital in Boston. I am fortunate in that I live about an hour away from Boston and, in my opinion, the home of some of the best hospitals in the world. The doctor that had done my ERCP recommended St Elizabeth's, Dana Farber Cancer Institute, and Mass General. I knew of a person that had been treated at St. Elizabeth's for pancreatic cancer five years ago, and he is now doing quite well. My son-in-law had been treated at Dana Farber/Brigham and Women's for Burkitt's Lymphoma and is also doing quite well. After a second person recommended Dana Farber, I decided that I would seek treatment there. My daughter, Kate, contacted her husband's doctor to get a recommendation as to who I should see at Dana Farber. Once all of those contacts had been made, I soon had a video conference with what would be my oncologist as well as my surgeon. I came to understand that Dana Farber is where you go to receive treatment for cancer, such as chemotherapy and radiation. However, if surgery is needed, then it is performed at Brigham and Women's, which is just across the street from Dana Farber. My trips to Dana Farber would begin a short time later when I went there for blood work, and a computerized tomography (CT) scan. This type of scan provides more information than an X-ray, and a dye would be used during a portion of my scan. Because of Covid, every time I entered Dana Farber, I had to go through a screening process that involved answering a series of Covid questions. Every time I went onto a different floor, I had to stop at a counter and go through the same set of Covid questions. Sometimes, within a 15-minute period, I would be asked basically the same questions three times. As I stood in line waiting to be processed, I would look at the other people there with me. Some looked healthy, but others looked like what you would think someone would look like if they were battling cancer. They were thin and bald or with hair that had been cropped shot. Some walked on their own, while others were in wheelchairs. Although there was a no-visitor policy, some had no choice but to have others with them to provide needed assistance. One thing I noticed immediately was that virtually no one made eye contact with anyone else. It was most difficult seeing young children, bald, in wheelchairs, and being pushed by their parents. I was 59 when I was diagnosed, which today is still considered young, but at least I had 59 good healthy years. Some of the kids that I encountered were maybe only 3 or 4. It is very difficult to see children having to go through this, having to fight this battle at such a young age. It is also very humbling.

After finally being cleared for blood work and my scan, I eventually found my way to the lab and imaging center. As I sat there, I texted my friend John. I noticed that many people were carrying backpacks or other bags filled with items to keep them occupied while they waited for whatever procedure they were having. I even remember taking a picture of some guy wearing nice new white sneakers and making some kind of joke or comment about them. Finally, a woman came into the room and said, "Mike F." I got up, and as I was walking toward her, she asked to see my hospital bracelet, which had been put on when I had registered earlier. I followed her to her office, and she asked me a series of questions regarding my visit for today. I was given my prep for the CT scan, which involved drinking two bottles of water over the next hour, one liter total. After completing this phase of the registration, I returned to the waiting area. After a short while, a nurse came out, called my name, checked my ID, and brought me back to her work space, where she started an IV and drew labs. When she was finished, I went back to the waiting area to slowly drink the water she had given to me. About an hour later, a technician came out, called my name, checked my ID, and brought me into the CT scanning room. I removed my shoes and everything that was in my pockets. I then lied down on the bed leading into the scan. They offered a warm blanket, and I accepted. My IV was connected to a dye that would later be pushed into my body. They told me that they would alert me before the dye went in. I was told to hold my arms over my head, and I had to keep them there for the duration of the scan. They then left the room, and I was given instructions over a speaker. I believe that the instructions are a recording because the voice, as well as the instructions, are the same every time. Basically, you are told to breath normally, then hold your breath, then breath again. This is repeated several times.

Finally, I was told that the dye was going to be injected. They told me that my body was going to get warm, and like a tough guy, like I think I am, I said to myself, "bring it;" well, they brought it. As the dye coursed through my body, I thought I was going to spontaneously combust. I got hot from head to toe. I could feel that my breath was warm, and it felt like my genitals were going to burst into flames at any time. I also got the feeling that I had to pee, which I figured I would use to extinguish the fire. The sensation dissipated in about 30 seconds, and the CT scan was now complete. The bed was removed from the CT scan, my IV was taken out, and I was done, just like that. I walked back to my car and drove home. I guess some of the good things about going through this during a pandemic are that there was not as much traffic in Boston, and I did not have to pay for parking.

By the time I got home, I had the results of my blood work and scans. Many of the things that were checked for in my blood were elevated, including my liver enzymes and my cancer markers. One specific cancer marker that was looked at was carbohydrate antigen 19-9 or just simply CA 19-9. CA 19-9 is a type of tumor marker made by cancer cells. High levels are often a sign of pancreatic cancer. The results of my scans were just as concerning; they seemed to show abnormalities everywhere. Besides the tumor in my pancreas, I had a large mass on the right side of my thyroid, spots in my liver and lungs, and an aneurysm on an artery leading to one of my kidneys, not to mention an adrenal adenoma which I had already known about. How does one cope with all of this? For me, the only thing I could do was put it all in my doctor's hands. It wasn't my problem; I gave all of my medical issues to my doctor. It was his responsibility to get me better, and I would do anything he told me to do. Although I am a firm believer that you must be an advocate of your own health, placing all of my healthcare needs in the hands of my physician allowed me the freedom to continue to "live my life." What was going to be was going to be, but I did not want to sit around and dwell on my condition. One thing that I did notice, which caused some questioning, was the fact that the scans taken at Dana Farber revealed that my pancreatic tumor was only around half the size of what I was told it was originally. This caused me to wonder about the results of other scans that I recently had back at home.

HOW WAS IT MISSED?

In September 2019, I went to my local emergency room and was diagnosed with kidney stones. Because I was told that the stone was very large and could not pass on its own, I was hospitalized overnight. By the morning, I felt fine but was told that I would have to wait another day in order to see a urologist. I began to think about what I was told regarding the size of the stone in question and realized that the stone was around 10 times smaller than what I was told. An error had been made in the conversion from centimeters to millimeters. I discussed this with my nurse and said that there was no reason for me to continue to stay in the hospital. I told her that I would come back if necessary and would also make an appointment to see my own urologist. A few weeks later, while visiting my urologist, he said, "you know you have an adrenal adenoma, right." I said apparently not, because I don't know what that is. He said, "I am going to make an appointment for you to see an endocrinologist." I came home and went and did a Google search for adrenal adenomas. I quickly found that an adrenal adenoma is a benign (noncancerous) mass located on top of the adrenal glands. I should have been happy with that explanation, but I kept searching and, of course, found the most sinister side possible. I was so caught up with my adrenal adenoma that I brought it up during my first discussion with my oncologist. I was almost more concerned about the adenoma than I was about the adenocarcinoma. Thinking about it, my oncologist must have thought that I was some kind of an idiot. Here I am more worried about something that is basically harmless versus something that is definitely going to kill me. Anyway, I saw an endocrinologist, and he ordered more blood work as well as another scan in March 2020. When I met with my endocrinologist in March, he said that the results of the scan showed that there was no change in the size of the adenoma. He also said that I have spinal degenerative disease. I thought great, one more thing to be concerned about. Less than a month later, I was diagnosed with a 4 cm mass in the head of my pancreas. The question that still haunts me is that in September and then again in March, I had scans of my abdominal cavity, and no one noticed a 4 cm mass in my pancreas?

REACHING OUT

I have, and continue to be, a very independent person. This can be viewed as a strength but also, at the same time, a weakness. There will always be times when we need the help of others, and people are willing to help, so let them. I recognized that I was going to need assistance, so I reached out to others, and their response was overwhelming. I had people offer to drive me to and from Boston, cut my lawn, deliver various types of food to my home and do my grocery shopping. I felt that if I ever needed something, all I had to do was reach out, and people would be there. My first experience with this was when my sister-in-law Betty drove me early in the morning to Brigham and Women's so that I could have my power port implanted in the right side of my chest. Through this port, I would receive all of my chemotherapy. It also allowed for blood to be drawn without the need for an additional needle stick. As always, I arrived early for my appointment. I actually went into the wrong building and had to be directed to the correct location. I remember sitting in a small waiting area completely alone. Finally, a set of double doors opened, and I was ushered inside a large room filled with hospital beds separated from each other by curtains. I was brought over to my bed, told to undress, and put on a hospital johnny. When I was finished, several nurses came over to me and began to ask me questions as we established a rapport. One nurse then started an IV in the back of my hand. I could see other patients that surrounded me. The nurses knew that I was there to have a port implanted and begin my treatment. One nurse pointed to a guy at the end of the room and said that he was there to have his port removed. I thought about him and prayed for the day when that would be me. I wondered what he had gone through, about the treatments that he endured. In the background, I could hear a nurse talking about a book she was reading by the author Jodi Picoult. I had read several books written by her and was curious as to which book the nurse was referring to. At one point prior to my procedure, a nurse looked at me and said that she was going to give me something to relax. I said to myself, I thought I was relaxed, but apparently, I must look nervous. Anyway, she did as she promised, and I guess I did feel more relaxed after receiving the medication. I think that she gave me a little Versed, now my drug of choice. After just a couple of milligrams, you can feel your body relax and just kind of sink into the bed. A doctor, or what I assume was a doctor, came over to me and explained the entire procedure and what I could expect afterward. I was told that I could bath immediately and, after a few days, even go swimming if I wanted. Shortly thereafter, I was wheeled into the operating room. I remember a nurse, probably a nurse anesthetist looking at me and saying, "You have nothing to worry about. I have a lot of drugs and am not afraid to use them." I guess she was telling the truth because I don't remember anything else about the procedure. I believe my time spent in the recovery room was brief. I also believe that Diane, my son-in-law's mother, along with my wife, brought me home. Again because of Covid, basically no one other than patients were allowed into the hospital. Prior to any procedure, contact information was obtained regarding the person who would be bringing that patient home. Once a procedure was complete, the person bringing the patient home was notified. Once that person arrived at the hospital, they would notify the hospital that they were there, and the patient would be wheeled out to the waiting vehicle. This same series of events would follow each of the five surgeries I had.

I don't believe that it took me long to recover from having my port implanted. I was seldom aware that I even had a port unless I looked at my chest in a mirror or I accidentally hit it against something. It was more of a psychological effect that bothered me. Every time I saw or felt it, I would be reminded of my condition, one in which, to some extent, I am a prisoner of my own disease. I have to do things that I really do not want to do. For example, once all of my treatments have been completed, I have to return to Dana Faber every three months for labs and every six months for a CT scan. I have to continue to do this for the next five years. It is not something I want to do, but I basically have no choice, and so sometimes I find myself getting up at 3:30 in the morning and leaving my house one hour later so that I can be on time for my appointment in Boston. I realize that I could probably have my labs and scans done locally, but by going to Dana Farber, I usually have all of my results by the time I get home. In my opinion, having that information available to me in a brief period of time is worth the ride to Boston. It is far better than dealing with the anxiety of waiting on test results.

ROUND 1 (4/28/20)

With my port in place, I was now ready to begin chemotherapy. The night prior to my first round of chemo, I remember feeling excited. I wanted to begin to fight back and destroy/kill that thing inside of me that was trying to kill me. I can't remember who had brought me to my first round of chemo, but prior to leaving my home, my wife put lidocaine cream on my skin, covering my port. The cream would serve to numb the area so that I would not feel the needle as it was inserted into my port. The skin over my port was free from hair as I had shaved the right side of my chest prior to the implantation of my port. Looking in the mirror, it looked kind of foolish, with only one side of my chest shaved, so I decided to shave my entire chest. That looked even more foolish with my chest bare but my abdomen with hair, so I shaved everything. When my ride finally arrived, I grabbed my back pack which contained a book, food and drink, my phone and charger, an extension cord, in case the power outlet was not near my bed, and a blanket. Once I have made my way inside of Dana Farber and past all of my check points, and have an ID bracelet placed around my wrist, I receive what I refer to as a tracking device that I must clip onto my clothing. Psychologically, the most difficult question to answer is when I am asked if I have a port, again, a constant reminder of my illness. I then walk over to the lab where my port will be accessed and blood drawn. The waiting area outside of the lab is kind of hard to describe. Actually, it is not the physical place itself but the people sitting there. No one makes eye contact; everyone just keeps to themselves. Some look healthy, while others do not so much. Some have a full head of hair, while others are bald or have their hair cropped short, or they are wearing a hat or skull cap. Nurses continuously come into the waiting room from behind closed doors and call out a person's first name, followed by their last initial. Once I heard the name Mike F called, I walked over to the nurse and showed her my ID bracelet. She leads me into her work-station, and I sit in a chair. The shirt I am wearing is a pull-over but has three buttons leading from the collar down. I undo the buttons in order to reveal my port. For some reason, I have to turn my head to the far left each time my port is accessed. Because of the lidocaine cream that I had applied earlier, I did not feel the needle pass through my skin and into my port. Once the needle is secured along with the Luer Lock and extension set, I head back to the elevators and make my way to the seventh floor. I have to check in just as I had done earlier, answering the exact same Covid questions and then sit in a waiting area to the left of the admittance counter. It is not long before a technician calls my name, checks my ID bracelet, and then proceeds to take my vital signs, including my pulse, blood pressure, temperature, and weight, and then back to the waiting area again. When called in again, I was led to a room where I was to meet with my oncologist nurse practitioner for the first time. I thought I was going to be seeing my doctor, but that was not the case. My nurse practitioner was extremely polite and professional and truly seemed to care. In fact, at one point, I thought that she was going to begin to cry. I actually looked at her and said that everything was going to be okay. She was quite thorough with her exam and explained things to me. When we were finished, I found myself again sitting in the waiting area, this time to the right of the admittance counter. After a brief while, my name was again called, and I was led to a room where I would be receiving chemo; the fun was about to begin. There were no beds in the room; instead, there was a recliner chair that faced a television. There were no windows and only a curtain separating me from the person next to me. When my nurse entered, she apologized for not having a room with a window view and said that she would try to have one for me during my next appointment. Like most everyone else there, including my nurse practitioner, she was much younger than I am; in fact, she was young enough to be my daughter. She asked if I wanted anything to eat or drink. Despite having brought food and drink with me, I accepted her offer and had a couple of snacks along with a vegetarian sandwich that came inside of a plastic bag. Once she had gotten me something to eat, she sat down next to me and explained everything that was going to be done and what I could expect from the side effects of the chemo. She was incredibly knowledgeable and comforting. I think we spoke for about an hour before she began my chemo. I don't remember everything she told me about many of my side effects until I began to experience them. Because I was receiving so much fluid, about two hours into my treatment, I had to pee quite frequently. I remember the first time I put my hand on the handle of the toilet, turned the knob on the sink faucet, and felt the water on my hands. It appeared to be unusually cold. There was also a pins and needles sensation in my fingertips whenever I touched something. My chemo treatment there lasted three and a half hours, and so once it started, I was able to contact the person that was going to pick me up and let them know the exact time they needed to be outside of Dana Farber. For the first chemo session, my friend Bobby went to my house, picked-up my wife, and arrived at Dana Farber at the exact time that I was ready to come home. Prior to me leaving, my nurse disconnected the chemo I was receiving there and then connected the chemo I would be getting at home through a small pump that I had to carry around with me for the next two days. All of the medications that my nurse gave me had to be double-checked by a second nurse before they could be administered.

When my nurse said that I was ready to leave, I simply got up with my pump inside of a case that was hung around my neck and left on my own accord. My head was in a fog, and anytime I touched something with my fingertips, it felt as though an electric shock was going through them. However, I had been back and forth to the bathroom many times and felt that I was quite safe to walk around and leave Dana Farber without any assistance. In fact, the thought of asking for assistance never occurred to me. Bobby was right on time and pulled up to the entrance of Dana Farber as I was walking out; it could not have been timed any better.

I was not nauseated or in any way did I feel sick; I was simply in a big head fog. I was always coherent with everything around me, but it always seemed like I was in a dream state. My wife, who was in the front passenger seat, got out of the car and sat in the back. She felt that I would be more comfortable sitting in the front. I told them about my experience that day, which made the trip back home seem relatively quick. I was not nauseated or uncomfortable; however, about a half hour into the ride, I needed to pee. I did not mention it to Bobby, and I know he would have stopped anywhere I wanted, but I just held it in and stopped talking. As we approached my home, I did tell Bobby that I had to pee, and he said that I should have said something earlier. As soon as we entered my driveway, I jumped out of the car and peed on the side of my lawn. It was dark out, so no one would be able to see me. I was anxious to get inside my home and have something to eat and then rest, but I went back over to the car and thanked Bobby for the ride home. He said that he would call me the following Wednesday and we would go out. I told him that it sounded like a great idea, thanked him again, and went into my house. My wife had made chicken soup, and I enjoyed a big bowl of it before retiring to the couch. Once on the couch, Bella, my 20-pound Basenji, would jump up and lie next to me, and I would cover us with a blanket. I then turned on the TV and put on the movie Jaws. Don't ask why, but I quickly fell asleep as soon as the movie was on. I never did see Chrissie get eaten by the shark. When I woke up, the credits were rolling up the screen. I then took Compazine to prevent nausea, as well as Xanax to help me sleep. Although I was also given Zofran, also for nausea, I was given a very large dose of it at Dana Farber and was told that I could not have any more for 48 hours.

The following day would be spent just lying around on the couch. Around 1:30, I would wash my hair in the kitchen sink and then take a shower from the waist down. I didn't want to get any water on my port now that I was receiving chemo, and I could not get my pump wet, so I would just hang the pump on the shower door and do the best I could to wash myself. Following my shower, I would go to bed and fall asleep. I slept for about three hours, and when I woke, I would have dinner in the kitchen before making my way back onto the couch. By 10 p.m., I was back in bed. Thursday and Friday were spent doing much the same. However, on Friday, around 5 p.m., after completing my chemo and shutting off my pump, my wife would remove the needle from my port and administer a shot of Neulasta into my arm. The Neulasta was used to increase my white blood cell count. I was told that it costs about $9,000.00 per injection. Thank goodness for insurance, for it only cost me $15. On Saturday morning, I was steroid high and felt pretty good. By the afternoon, I was tired and needed to rest. I think Sunday was my worst day because I was very fatigued. I have made a distinction between being tired and being fatigued. When I was tired, I could sleep, but when I was fatigued, I did not feel like doing anything. Sometimes I would sit for an hour on the edge of the couch, looking at a blank TV screen. I just did not feel like doing anything, but I was also not tired, so I could not sleep. On Monday, I was in a head fog. I tried to be a little more active and would spend a few minutes on my elliptical or shooting baskets in my driveway. Tuesday found me feeling slightly better but still not all that well. Sometime during the afternoon, while lying on the couch, I received a phone call from Bobby, who asked me if I was ready for him to pick me up the following day. I really wasn't feeling very well, but I succumbed to peer pressure and said that I was. When I hung up the phone, I thought to myself, what am I thinking about? I still feel like "shit." I laid back down and tried to get myself psychologically ready to go out.

THE PUMP

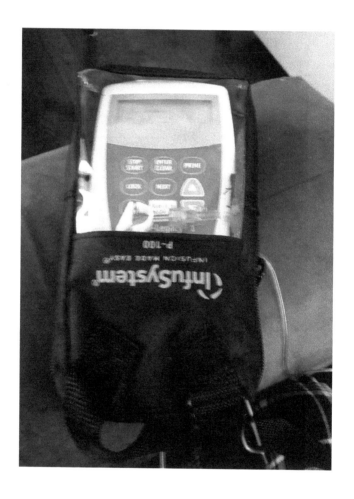

TAKE ME FOR A WALK

On Wednesday, I got out of bed, took a shower, and prepared myself for my outing. Bobby showed up promptly at 10 a.m. He drove to a state reservation, where we went for a walk. At one point, he stumbled on roots and nearly fell. I said to myself, who is the one who is supposed to be weak and sick here. The walk was fantastic, and although tired, it felt great to be outside doing something. Once we were finished, we went to a pizza shop and ordered roast beef subs. Following chemo, I had a huge craving for red meat. Normally my diet consisted of fruits, vegetables, fish, and chicken. I was not much of red meat eater. However, at one point, while taking a shower, I felt very hungry, and a piece of lettuce was just not going to cut it. In fact, I did not even feel like eating chicken or fish, I needed red meat, and I did not care what kind it was. That is when I started ordering roast beef subs and then later just purchasing roast beef from the supermarket and making my own. Anyway, once Bobby and I purchased our subs, we went back to Bob's condo and ate them. We talked for a little while after that, and he then brought me home. When I got home, I was tired but felt so much better. Bobby would continue to do this every Wednesday following chemo. However, instead of walking in the woods, we would walk at Cherry and Webb Beach in Westport, MA. We would walk the beach for about two miles each time. After our walk, we would then order and eat Hawaiian pizza back at his condo. Throughout my entire treatment, I believe that there were only two times when he was not available, and so my friends Joe and Rick stepped in for him. I honestly believe that this day was a game changer for me, and I began to refer to it as my turn around day. On Thursday, I began to cycle and would ride for about 7 miles; and then on Friday, I would up that milage to 14. I rode 14 miles every day until the following Wednesday, chemo day. During that time period, I would ride over 70 miles and walk another 6. I needed to regain my strength before my next round of chemo. I envisioned it like being in the ring with Mike Tyson; you knew you were going to get your ass kicked, but I felt that maybe I could run around the ring for a little while and get a few punches in before the knockout blow came; it was better than just standing there, doing nothing but getting beaten up.

THE PARADE

On Tuesday afternoon, May 12, 2020, I was about to receive a huge surprise, one that I would be eternally grateful for. Just prior to my second round of chemo, my oldest daughter, along with her husband, and my youngest daughter, along with her future husband, visited me at my home. We were in the kitchen standing around and talking, when my older daughter suggested that we go outside. I walked out the back door and onto my deck. We hung out there talking until my younger daughter asked to see the new net that I had just placed on my basketball hoop. At first, I thought this request somewhat strange, but I said OK. We walked through the house and back out the front door, where we just kind of stood in the driveway. I think the guys might have gotten a basketball and were shooting around. While this was happening, I heard sirens. Every time I hear sirens, I usually say, "well, gotta go," as it is often an ambulance that I am hearing, and being a paramedic, I often respond to many of these emergencies. I remember one such instance, while planning to go out and celebrate my daughter's birthday, the sound of sirens prompted me to respond to my neighbor's home to help deliver a baby. As my neighbor was lying on her front lawn, I remember waiting for the ambulance to arrive as the baby had just been delivered. Having the same birth date as my daughter made it extra special.

The sirens became louder as they approached my house. I soon saw emergency lights turn down the street just prior to my own. As I continued to watch, something did not seem quite right. The vehicles, although traveling at a constant speed, were not going very fast. As they rounded the corner, I realized what was happening. They were not responding to an emergency but were leading a parade of vehicles that would soon pass my home in support of me. The parade lasted for nearly 15 minutes as around 100 vehicles drove past me. There were police cars, ambulances and fire trucks, and other support vehicles from the Towns of Mattapoisett and Rochester, as well as from the City of New Bedford. There was also a State Police cruiser. Among these emergency vehicles were horn-honking cars filled with friends and family, many of them colleagues from New Bedford High School. I believe I even saw a few former students. Some had their cars decorated and #Floriostrong written on their windows. They were holding balloons and waving poster boards, wishing me well. They even had FUN 107, a local radio station, play music during that time in my honor. It was a true display of friendship and support. It made me feel as though I was not in this battle alone, that together we would be victorious. Even months later, the #Floriostrong could still be seen on some vehicles.

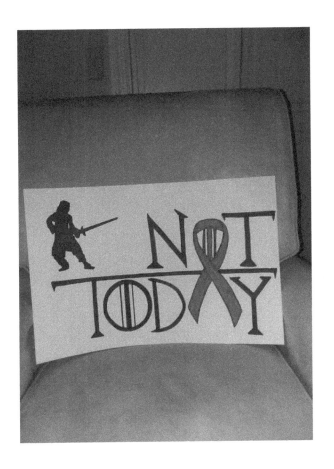

MONETARY SUPPORT

What followed were monetary donations from the Rochester Fire Department and New Bedford Emergency Medical Services. One individual from New Bedford Emergency Medical Services donated what I consider a large sum of money. He said he was giving back to me that which I had given him while he was my student at New Bedford High. When I began teaching at New Bedford High

School in 2004, I started and implemented an Emergency Medical Technician (EMT) program in the school. Students could take and EMT class as an elective in their course selection. Those that successfully completed the class, could then opt to become certified as an EMT by passing a State or National exam. The exam consisted of a written portion as well as a practical session. This particular student became certified as an EMT and is now a paramedic working for the City of New Bedford. He indicated that at the time when he was eligible to take his exam, he did not have the money to pay for it, so I gave him the money so he could take the exam. Truthfully, although I know that I had done that for some students, I don't actually remember paying for him. As a teacher, you just do things for kids without ever considering any type of reciprocity. This student truly paid it forward. In fact, he pays it forward every time he responds to 911 emergencies and renders care to the sick and injured.

I would be remiss if I did not mention that despite the very generous donation made by the Rochester Fire Department, they also, at one point, dropped off several clam dinners they had left over from one of their clam bakes – they were truly appreciated.

ROUND TWO (5/13/20)

Right now, I am having my second round of chemo at Dana-Farber. It has been over a month since I was diagnosed with pancreatic cancer on April 9th. I am fortunate enough to be able to get rides to and from the facility; thanks to all my friends and family, in that regard, at least the price of gas in down.

Because of Covid, traffic is light coming into Boston. Also, because of Covid, parking at Dana-Farber is free, but that doesn't really matter because the only people allowed inside are patients. I was dropped off at the front door around 10 a.m. and will be ready to be picked up around 4:45 p.m. Again, I am fortunate enough to have one person drop me off and another pick me back up.

Once I arrive and pass through three Covid screening check points I will encounter, I go to the lab where blood is drawn through the port in my chest. Having them access the port is a lot easier than starting an IV each time, but it is still slightly uncomfortable. Unfortunately, today my port was blocked, so the blood had to be drawn via a needle stick. They put an enzyme into the port, and it is now working fine.

Once labs are drawn, I meet with my nurse practitioner. By the time I have that meeting, the results of my labs have come back and are evaluated and discussed between us. After the meeting is over and I have been examined, I again have to check in and wait to be called for my treatment. I am then brought in to a room where I sit in a recliner which is heated and can provide a massage. My nurse attaches me to chemo. The run lasts for 3.5 hours. When finished, I will be sent home with a pump that delivers another 46 hours of chemo. On Friday, I can shut off the pump, flush out and remove the line leading into the port inside of my chest. My wife will then give me a shot of Neulasta, a medication that helps increase my white blood cell count. This process will continue every other week for the next three months. It will be followed by a week of radiation and then surgery. I hope to be cancer free by Thanksgiving. It may seem like a long road, but "it is what it is," and you "do what you gotta do."

A Letter to My Cancer by Ginger Johnson, which I modified slightly.

IT MAY SEEM LIKE YOU HAVE CONTROL OF MY LIFE RIGHT NOW BUT YOU REALLY DON'T. YOUR PRESENCE ONLY MAKES ME STRONGER, BRAVER, KINDER, WISER. I CAN CHOOSE HOW I THINK, WHAT I SPEAK, AND HOW I LOVE. YOU WILL NEVER BE ABLE TO TOUCH THOSE THINGS, NEVER.

May 14, 2020

Just a brief follow-up from yesterday. My chemo ended at 4:30 p.m. exactly 3.5 hours from when it began. I was connected to my 46 hours of take-home chemo via a pump, which only takes seconds to do. Because of the atropine I am given during my infusion, my pupils become dilated, which I am sure accounted for the blurred vision that I recall having after my first session. During the last 30 minutes of my treatment, I have to pee frequently. I know that the word urinate is probably more appropriate, but I like the work pee better. The problem with the frequent urge to urinate is the hour-plus ride home. Now with Covid, good luck in finding a public restroom open. I stopped at the bathroom located in the visitors center of the Blue Hills, but it was closed, and the State Police would not let me use their facility either, so I had my friend stop at one of the trail heads at the Blue Hills. I walked down the trail until I was kind of out of sight and went behind a large tree. Now there was no one else around when I started to go, but as fate with have it, no sooner did I start peeing when a man began to walk down the same trail. I normally would interrupt myself and stop the flow in midstream; yes, I have done this before, but at that moment, when you are not really feeling all that well, I did not care, and would apologize to him as he passed by. However, when he saw me, he stopped and acted as a true gentleman allowing me my privacy. I thanked him and apologized as he later passed by. I believe that most people are inherently descent and kind. I view people as being intelligent, always willing to learn, knowing that they don't know everything, and either changing or solidifying their beliefs as new knowledge is obtained. Yet, I also believe that there are those that you might say are just ignorant and not willing to do any of those things. Unfortunately, you will encounter them as well. I try not to get angry with these people when I do encounter them, or at least not to take that anger with me. It is said that holding onto anger is like drinking poison and expecting the other person to die. I came across something which read like this. If you had $86,400 in and account and someone stole $10 from you, would you be upset and throw all the remaining $86,390 away in hopes of getting back at the person who took your $10, or would you just move on with your life? We have 86,400 seconds each day. Don't let someone's negative 10 seconds ruin the remaining 86,390. Life is much more precious than that.

When I arrived back home, I had a wonderful meal waiting for me that a friend had dropped off; thank you very much. After stuffing myself, I made my way to the couch and turned on the TV mostly for background noise. Because of the steroids I was given, I was told that I would not be able to sleep, but I was tired and feel asleep for about 45 minutes. I woke up feeling miserable, another learning experience because I can't describe it other than that. I had no pain or discomfort anywhere. I was not nauseated and had no headache or fever. I just felt lousy. Other side effects that I experienced immediately after treatment are pins and needles in my fingertips, especially when I touched something cold. Also, that same sensation occurred on my tongue following putting something cold in my mouth. When I swallowed a liquid or something cold, it felt as though it was stuck in the back of my throat. The last time these sensations subsided over the next few days, and I am hoping the same will occur this time.

ROUND THREE (5/27/20)

Today, I began my third round of chemotherapy. I was dropped off at the main entrance to Dana-Farber, 450 Brookline Ave. Upon exiting the vehicle, I thanked my friend for the ride and closed the car door. I wanted to turn and wave or at least watch him pull away, but my focus was on the automatic door entrance to a place that I never dreamed I would pass. Once inside, I proceed to the right and stand in line. There are marks on the floor indicating where a person should stand, maintaining social distancing, a term we have all become too familiar with. I look at the people standing around me, all wearing masks, and realize that they have or had cancer. Either way, they are all cancer patients. Some look healthier than others, but no one seems to or wants to make eye contact with anyone else. So, we all stand in silence as we wait to be registered, and it is only at the "check-in" points that you hear people speak as they answer yes or no to a battery of Covid questions; their monotone voice indicates frustration.

Once I have passed my first round of questioning, I take the elevator to the second floor, where the lab is located. Some of the people that were there with me on the first floor are also here standing in line, waiting to be "checked-in" again and answer their second round of Covid questions, the same as just minutes before. In the lab, my port is accessed, and blood is drawn; I am now ready for chemo. I take the elevator to the 7th floor and get "checked-in" on that floor, again answering the same

Covid questions for my final time. I am called into a room, my vital signs are taken, and I am again sent back into the waiting area. The next time I am called back in, I meet with my nurse practitioner. Once that meeting is over, I am sent back out only to have to be "checked-in" again so that I can begin chemo. At least at this final "check-in," they spared me the Covid questions. I am then brought into another area where I receive my chemo. The chemo has to be specially ordered and is not ready until after I arrive. Once the chemo has started, it takes exactly 3.5 hours to run.

This is all a very tedious process, and if not for the tremendous amount of support I receive from family and friends, it would be nearly impossible to do; I cannot that you enough. In particular, I would not be able to go through this without my wife. She is with me 24/7, advocating for me with guidance and encouragement. Protecting me from becoming ill, especially during these times, by disinfecting every item that comes into our home. A bottle of hand sanitizer is kept right at our front door.

ROUND FOUR (6/10/20)

Today, I begin my fourth round of chemotherapy for pancreatic cancer; I am halfway there. Following four more treatments, I will begin radiation therapy, followed by surgery. I am still plagued with abdominal discomfort every day. I am hoping that this feeling will eventually go away; I have had it for around 10 weeks already, and it is very tiresome and discouraging. I often feel that this will be my new normal and just something I will have to deal with – I hope not. On the brighter side, I have not been sick from the chemo and have had very little nausea and no vomiting. I have never lost my appetite and even gained a few pounds. My hair loss has been minimal, and with the exception of the Wednesday on which I receive chemo, I have been able to sleep without difficulty. I have developed chemotherapy-induced peripheral neuropathy, a side effect of the chemo, in which my fingertips experience a pins and needles sensation, especially when in contact with something cold. That sensation is also felt on my tongue and throat anytime when in contact with cold food or drink. These symptoms develop very shortly after beginning chemo, and although they diminish with time, they last for nearly two weeks or until the next treatment, when they begin all over again.

ANOTHER CAT SCAN

On June 18th, I am scheduled for another CAT Scan. The scan takes only minutes to do and is not really that bad. My body is scanned from my neck down to my lower abdomen. I can leave clothes on, but I make certain that there is nothing in my pockets. I can even leave my watch on as my arms are held over my head and do not enter the scanner itself. Once in the room, I lie on my back on a table, which can be remotely moved into and out of the CAT scanner. A device holding the dye is attached to my port. The staff have always been kind and considerate and covered me with a warm blanket. Once ready to go, I am left in the room alone. A recorded message tells me when to breathe as well as when to hold my breath. After being moved into and out of the scanner several times, I was told that the dye would now be pushed into my port. Again, this makes my body hot. Even my breath is hot, and I feel the urge to pee, but because I have gone through this before, I am ready for all of these sensations. Once the scans are complete, the device containing the dye is removed from my port, and I am allowed to leave. I am only slightly lightheaded when I sit up but otherwise, fine. I am advised to drink a lot of water to help flush out the dye. I don't like having to do this. I don't like the fact that some kind of dye is traveling through my blood stream. I don't like the fact the chemo is also doing the same thing. I often think about what the long-term effects of all of my treatments will be and realize that I have no other choice. I guess I should be grateful if I live long enough for me to be affected by long-term side effects; many do not.

I was watching Rocky Balboa the other day. The following comes from a speech he gave to his son.

"The world ain't all sunshine and rainbows, it's a very mean and nasty place, and I don't care how tough you are. It will beat you to your knees and keep you there permanently if you let it. You, me, or nobody is going to hit you as hard as life. But it ain't about how hard you hit. It's about how hard you can get hit and keep moving forward. How much you can take and keep moving forward. That's how winning is done."

That is how I am going to win and defeat cancer. No matter what is thrown at me, I am going to press on and keep moving forward.

June 13, 2020

In life, things often do not go as planned, such as what happened today. Following my 46 hours of chemo, which I receive via an infusion pump while at home, I am given an injection of Neulasta. This medication increases my white blood cell count to a level about twice as high as normal. Raising my white blood cell count, in particular neutrophils, decreases the chances of getting and infection. Normally, I pick-up my Neulasta at the pharmacy at Dana-Farber. However, this week, because my chemo treatment began and ended later than usual, by the time I went to the pharmacy, it was closed. I notified my doctor's office of the situation, and they contacted the pharmacy. I was told that I should receive it by 10:30 Friday morning. By 3 p.m. the medication had still not arrived. I found out that it had been shipped via UPS. I contacted UPS and was informed that it would not arrive at my house until around 3 PM on Monday. I explained to UPS that I needed the medication now and that Monday would be too late. I also explained to them that the medication has to be refrigerated, and the cost for the two doses being sent to me is about $18,000. They basically told me that they were sorry and would do the best they could. Because of this set-back, I had to make a special trip to Dana-Farber to receive a 5-second injection. As I have always stated, "You do what you gotta do." The medication finally arrived on Wednesday. On my next visit to Dana-Farber, I returned this medication to the pharmacy, and I believe they just disposed of it.

June 15, 2020

On this date, I share a few thoughts on how I feel both mentally and physically. Opening up and sharing with you helps me cope with what I have to go through. I know that some people like to keep things to themselves, but I would rather discuss it.

On April 9th, my diagnosis date, I thought the worst and began to get some of my personal affairs in order. I remember hearing that pancreatic cancer was one of the worst cancers you could get. It is painful and has a high mortality rate.

Every day for nearly two months, I have had a stomach ache or other forms of abdominal pain, and chemo presents with its own side effects. Right now, the days following chemo are the worst. The steroids make me shaky and tired. It takes almost a week before those side effects go away. However, the pain and abdominal discomfort that I have experienced for the last two months have diminished significantly, and I feel much better.

I spend most of the days following chemo just resting, but as I begin to feel better, I begin exercising to regain my strength. After my third round of chemo, I walked a total of 7 miles and cycled 41. I was also able to open my pool and cut nearly the acre of lawn that my house sits on. I am regaining weight, have never felt nauseated or otherwise sick, never lost my appetite or hair, and my skin color is good. In fact, when I walk into Dana-Farber, I feel like I don't belong there. I have responded well to treatment. All of my lab work is mostly within normal range, and those that are not are not far off.

This Thursday, June 18th, I will have another CT scan as well as a biopsy of the nodule on my thyroid. On June 24th, my next chemo date, and my daughter Kate's birthday, I will meet with my doctor to review the results of my CT scan and the biopsy, and discuss future treatment plans.

I recognize that I still have a long fight ahead of me, and there will be times when I am not feeling as good as I would like to. However, in general, I feel quite well both mentally and physically. This has been and will continue to be a life-altering experience, one that, in the end, will make me a much better person with greater compassion and understanding of other people's needs and struggles.

Sometimes you have to let go of the picture of what you thought life would be like and learn to find joy in the story you are actually living. (Rachel Marie Martin)

June 19, 2020

I wish I did not know this...

Dana-Farber Cancer Institute, the Yawkey Center, is located at 450 Brookline Ave, Boston. There is a parking garage just beyond the main entrance, which because of Covid, is for patients only and is free of charge. When you enter the garage, you go down to the 3rd level and park anywhere. An elevator brings you to the lobby. (There is a bathroom located on level 1 of the garage) Another set of elevators, located in the lobby, or first floor, will take you anywhere else in the building. Located on the second floor are the labs where you go for blood work. The pharmacy can also be found on that floor. The third floor is where the cafeteria and garden are located. It is also where you will find the sky bridge that brings you to the other building, which is across the street from the Yawkey Center. It is in this building where all the imagining, like CAT scans, is done. Once you enter this building, take the elevator, easily located, to L-1, and the entrance to imaging is right outside the elevator. The other floors of Yawkey Center are designated for various different types of cancer treatments. My type of cancer is treated on the 7th floor.

I wish I did not know any of this, but I do.

Yesterday I returned to Boston for a biopsy of the nodule on my thyroid as well as for a CAT scan of my chest, abdomen, and pelvis. It took seven and a half hours from the time I left my house until the time I returned. The biopsy of the nodule was performed at Brigham and Women's Hospital, which is only a block away from Dana-Farber. Interestingly enough, their imaging center is also located on Level L-1. A technician first performed an ultrasound of my thyroid, and then I met with the endocrinologist who did the biopsy. The endocrinologist first examined me and asked me a series of questions as well as allowed me to ask my own. She then explained the entire procedure and what I could expect. Once she was done, an entire team of doctors, at least four and all female, entered the room, and the biopsy was taken. A local anesthetic was injected into my neck. I believe a need was inserted into three different areas of my neck and into the nodule. The entire process lasted no more than five minutes and was relatively painless.

The CAT scan, done back at Dana-Farber, was also relatively painless. My port had to be accessed because a dye was used during the scan. I now prepare myself for the "hot sensation" caused by the dye, so it doesn't bother me as much.

In about a week, I should have the results of my biopsy. If it is cancerous, then I will have surgery to remove it. I was told that even if it was cancerous and then removed, no further treatment would be needed.

June 23, 2020

It is a big day for me tomorrow. I will meet with my oncologist to discuss my test results and future plans. It is also my last scheduled chemo, although I believe I have another three.

There are various forms of chemo specifically designed to treat different types of cancer and delivered in a variety of different ways. They all produce side effects that vary from person to person. Each time I asked my oncologist or nurse practitioner if I would experience a certain side, their response was always the same; you may or may not.

The following are the side effects I have experienced. I have sort of broken them down by the frequency in which they occur.

Side effects I get all the time.

Pins and needles in fingers, tongue, and throat when in contact with cold.

Shakiness.

Cracked corners of my mouth.

Difficulty swallowing due to the lack of saliva. This was followed by drooling and sometimes choking on my own saliva.

Side effects I get often.

Acid reflux.

Burps.

Hiccups.

Fatigue.

Tiredness.

Weakness.

Feeling foggy.

Feeling stoned.

Don't feel right.

Dots that float past my visual field – not floaters

Some difficulty either falling asleep or staying asleep.

Side effects I have experienced once.

Painful hiccups.

TMJ (temporomandibular joint dysfunction) or at least what I call TMJ. I would have severe pain at the angle of my jaw when I first began to chew something. That feeling would dissipate the more I chewed.

A hot flash. It felt as though my entire body was on fire, and I had to remove my clothing. Good thing I was alone at home.

Sores on the roof of my mouth.

Common side effects that I have only minimally experienced.

Hair loss.

Nausea.

Sided effects that have been experienced by others that I have never experienced.

Vomiting.

Loss of appetite.

ROUND FIVE (6/24/20)

Today was the first time I met with my oncologist. All the other times, I have met with my nurse practitioner. There was nothing really different that came out of my meeting with him versus with my NP, and although he is not a bad-looking guy, my NP is a lot cuter. My CAT scan revealed that my tumor had shrunk slightly. Also, the stent that had been placed in my bile duct has shifted slightly but does not appear problematic. My lab values from my blood work are also good. The cancer marker CA19-9 has now come down to 66. The normal high is 34. The highest I have been was 135. To kind of put that into perspective, my doctor stated that we will see patients today, in which that marker will be several hundred thousand; I'll take 66.

Right now, my future plans include three more rounds of chemo followed by another CAT scan. If it all looks okay at that point, then radiation every day for five days. A month later, around October, I will have Whipple surgery. During this surgery, the head of my pancreas, where the tumor is located, will be removed. Also, my duodenum, the first part of my small intestine, will also be removed along with my gallbladder. Then, my stomach and pancreas will be reattached to a lower portion of my small intestine. I understand that the surgery could last anywhere from 8 – 12 hours. I will probably remain in the hospital for one week. It could take up to two months to completely recover.

The biopsy of my thyroid came back as undetermined significance, meaning that they are not sure if it is cancerous or not. Therefore, on July 2nd, I will have another biopsy at Brigham and Women's. They do not want to do surgery if it is not cancerous. If it is cancerous, then half of my thyroid will be removed. The surgery will be done as an outpatient procedure.

My oncologist appeared pleased with my progress and with the amount of exercise I am getting. I was able to cycle 72 miles after my last round of chemo. I was told by my nurse that exercise helps to diminish the effect of chemo. Looking forward to next week when I will feel well enough again to get back out there.

On a personal note, to myself, I realize that it really sucks that I have cancer. However, there are so many people at Dana-Farber that I believe are much worse off than I am, and so I am fortunate in that regard. I am also fortunate to have so many people in my corner offering me support at so many different levels.

July 1, 2020

Both yesterday and today, I had a video conference with two different doctors from the radiology department at Dana-Farber. They were extremely kind and considerate and appeared to be generally concerned with my health condition. They were also both pleased with my current treatment and the way I have responded to that treatment. My tumor has shrunk considerably due to chemo. Of concern to them is whether my tumor has any vascular involvement with any type of vein or artery, in particular with arterial involvement. I was told that although the vein might be against the tumor, the tumor is not wrapped around it, and there is no arterial involvement which will make surgery much easier.

My last chemo is slated for August 5th. On August 3rd or 4th, I will undergo radiation mapping, and on August 19th, I will begin radiation therapy. The idea of the radiation is to shrink the tumor even more than it is. I now believe that I am correct in thinking that the chemo is used to kill or destroy my cancer cells, and the radiation will be used to further shrink the tumor. The radiation I will be receiving will be done with the use of an MRI. Most radiation, or at least the form that I will be receiving, is done under a CAT scan. Dana-Farber is one of 10 institutions in the country that uses an MRI. They feel that this is a better and safer way to deliver this type of radiation therapy. Each treatment will take about an hour. I will undergo 5 consecutive days of treatment. A month following radiation, I will have surgery. Then for the next five years, I will have follow-up examinations at Dana-Farber every three months.

My reflection on this day includes the following:

Boston, Massachusetts, harbors some of the best hospitals in the world. Many of them are research and teaching hospitals, with students coming from a variety of institutions, including Harvard Medical School. Although driving to Boston can be somewhat stressful, it takes less than an hour and a half to get there, and I feel comfortable and confident in the care I am receiving. This experience has taught me to live more in the moment and appreciate and enjoy the simple things in life. Even eating an ice cream cone seems to have more meaning, bringing more enjoyment as a savor the flavor more than I did in the past; so what if it begins to melt, that is what napkins are for, just put it in a cup.

Ten years from now, someone is going to mention pancreatic cancer, and my ears are going to "perk up," and I am going to say, "Oh yeah, pancreatic cancer, I had that once."

One day you will thank yourself for not giving up (Unknown)

ROUND SIX (7/8/20)

I am now in my sixth round of chemo. I can't believe that I have been in this battle for over 3.5 months. I am no longer just optimistic but positive that in a short time, I will be cancer free. I still have two more rounds of chemo before radiation and then surgery. I admit that I am slightly anxious about radiation and slightly nervous about the surgery, but I will get through it just as I have done with chemo.

I feel lucky that things have gone the way they have; it could have been a lot worse. Although every day I experience some type of pain or discomfort, those symptoms have decreased in intensity and duration. I still recognize that there are a lot of people far sicker than I have ever been. Besides being terminal, many people will receive some form of treatment their entire life; for me, I am just passing through this thing called cancer and hope I never have to endure this type of fight again.

It is said that we cannot control the fruits of our actions. What you do or say can influence others in ways that you could never imagine. Even the simplest things could alter a person's life. My daughter Mikayla gave me a small wooden box to me, and on the box, it reads, "You Got This." My wife placed the box in an area that I frequently pass; I see it and read it often. That message, as simple as it is, has given me strength in times when I have needed it.

I would say that 99% of the time, I am content, not depressed or feeling down; last night before I went to bed was not one of those times. Knowing what I am facing today, I took my dog out for a short walk, all the while thinking that I don't want to do this anymore – chemo. It makes me feel horrible, and I cannot do the things I want to do for an entire week thereafter. I even pause in my yard before going into my house for reflection. Then just before retiring for the evening, I checked my phone for messages and noticed that there was one from a person that I had recently been in contact with but hadn't seen in years. The message read, "Good luck tomorrow." The entire way I had been feeling prior to reading that message changed in an instant. You see, the person who sent it has cancer and has undergone radiation and has been on chemo for years, and will continue to receive it for the rest of her life. After today, I have only two more sessions left. So, I feel lucky, for I am in a better state than many others. The fruits of the message she sent changed my entire demeanor. I went to bed peacefully and contented. *(In memory of Ann Collins, a true warrior, thank you)*

God grant me the serenity to accept the things I cannot change, the courage to change the things I can, and the wisdom to know the difference.

ROUND 7 (7/22/20)

One more round to go and then 5 days of radiation beginning August 19th, followed by surgery 4 to 6 weeks later. Once the tumor is removed, it will be analyzed in order to determine if more chemo is needed.

It is hard to believe that I have been doing this for about 4 months; it is still not any easier. Although I physically feel better and have gained weight, the side effects of chemo have not changed. It still takes me a full week before I feel somewhat normal and begin to resume regular activities. This is a little frustrating because as time went on, I thought I would adjust and begin to feel better quicker. Along with the frustration, and feeling better overall, I have moments when I have begun to feel "mad" that all of this has happened to me. This is not a negative feeling, or one of anger, but one of motivation for me to do more and fight harder. It is a burning desire to continue to forge forward in my treatment process. To do whatever has to be done to eventually put this nightmare behind me.

I have placed my trust entirely in the hands of my medical team, and will do whatever they tell me; while at the same time realizing that I must always advocate for myself, making sure that I am receiving to best care and treatment possible. Even though they, my medical team, are experts in their field, I am not afraid to "speak out" so that my concerns are addressed.

My latest CA 19-9 level was 39. There normal high value for this pancreatic enzyme marker is 34; I am only 5 points away. I initially started at 135. As previously stated before, some people are in the hundreds of thousands.

I am looking forward to August 5th, my last chemo treatment at this time. Besides the side effects from chemo that I have already mentioned, the corners of my mouth remain constantly cracked. Other side effects, which resolved prior to my next chemo, include: My tongue turns white and somewhat painful. My throat becomes sore, and there is some discomfort when swallowing food. A smooth film, the best I can describe it, coats my teeth and mouth.

I received the result of the second biopsy of the nodule on my thyroid. It has been determined that the nodule remains suspicious for being cancerous. This means that there is a 50/50 chance that it is cancerous. Therefore, I will need surgery to remove the nodule and half of my thyroid. The surgery is outpatient, meaning I will be home the same day. Once the nodule is removed, it will be further analyzed for a diagnosis of whether it is cancerous or not. If it is cancerous, the entire thyroid will have to be removed. I will complete all of my pancreatic cancer treatments before having surgery on my thyroid.

August 1, 2020

Nearly 2 million people in the United States are diagnosed with some type of cancer each year. Your chances of developing cancer in your lifetime are almost 40%. Those are high numbers, and my hopes are that all of you will be in the 60% bracket that never has to face this dreadful disease.

I am sharing my journey with you so that you have an understanding of what it is like for someone living with and being treated for cancer. There are millions of other journeys, but this one is mine.

I have now completed 7 rounds of chemo, and am experiencing its' cumulative effects. I have started to lose some of my hair, the corners of my mouth are constantly cracked, there is always a tingling sensation in my fingers, and my hands are shaky. Even though this Wednesday is my last scheduled chemo treatment, I dread going. I feel pretty good right now and will continue to get better over the next few days. A week from now, I will be laid up on the couch again. As I feel better physically, I feel worse mentally because of my awareness of what is to come next week.

Whenever you find yourself doubting how far you can go, just remember how far you have come. Remember everything you have faced, all the battles you have won, and all the fears you have overcome! (Unknown)

On Monday, I will return to Boston for radiation mapping as I prepare for stage II of my journey. I still don't know what radiation mapping entails, but I will inform you when I do. I can tell you that I have to prepare for it. Every day for the past week, I had to take MiraLAX once a day and Gas X four times a day. According to my wife, the Gas X is not working, and all this time, I thought she wore a mask to prevent me from getting Covid.

August 3, 2020

So those of you that stated that radiation mapping was not that big of a deal were right. The process was relatively painless. I first met with a nurse who accessed my port. I then went for a CT scan. While lying on the CT scan, I was given a small amount of water to drink. At some point during the scan, a dye was injected into me via my port. Like before, the dye caused me to get hot. My hot breath, blowing back on my face because of the mask I was wearing, exacerbated this condition. During part of the CT scan, I had to practice holding my breath. I had to do this several times. Apparently, they can monitor how much air I take in each time I hold my breath. They want that amount of air relatively consistent each time. Once the CT scan was complete, I received my tattoos. A small dot was left on each side of my body and one on my abdomen. To make the dots/tattoos, a small amount of ink is injected just under my skin. The procedure is relatively painless.

After I was marked, I went for an MRI. All of my radiation will be done with the help of an MRI. As stated before, Dana-Farber is only one of ten institutions in the country that utilizes an MRI to assist with radiation therapy. By using an MRI, the radiation can be given more accurately, which causes less damage to surrounding tissues and organs. Most other institutions utilize a CT scan during radiation which does not offer the same benefits as an MRI.

The MRI I went into today had a tube as long as my body. Before the MRI, I was again given a small amount of water to drink. I was then strapped down to prevent me from moving and given hearing protection. I am not claustrophobic, so none of this presented as a problem. A mirror was placed in front of me so that when I looked into it, I could see a TV monitor in the back of me. During radiation, the monitor is going to allow me to see how deeply I breathe just prior to holding my breath. By using the monitor as a guide, I should be able to take in the same amount of air each time I am instructed to hold my breath. My 5 days of radiation treatment will begin on August 19th and end on August 25th; no radiation over the weekend. Each treatment should last about one hour.

So, there you have it. The mapping process was basically painless, with no noticeable side effects.

Hopefully, the last chemo is this Wednesday; I can't wait to be done with that.

ROUND EIGHT (8/5/20)

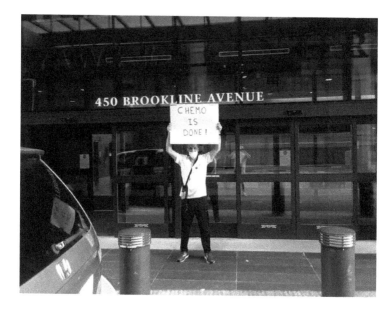

As you can see, I am still receiving chemo through my take-home pump. That will be removed on Friday at 4:30. It feels great, however, not to have to return to Dana-Farber for any more chemo until perhaps after surgery, which will be in about 2 months. Once the tumor is removed and analyzed, then a determination will be made if more chemo is needed. Until that time, I will continue to feel better and stronger.

On September 9th, I meet in person with my Surgeon. He made it clear that it had to be an in-person visit vs. a virtual conference.

As I stood there on that August 5th day, holding that sign over my head, I was met by cheers from onlookers and honking horns. Although I knew that the effects from this round of chemo would last for a week, I felt elated that this could be my last chemo treatment. I hate chemo. It is just so draining on the body. Following all the photo shoots, and just prior to getting into my friend's car, I encountered another individual standing outside of Dana Farber. Today was his first round of chemo for the same type of cancer I have. We talked briefly, and my heart went out to him. I felt as though we had an immediate bond. I knew nothing of his past, not even his name, but I knew something of his future and the battle that he was fighting. He remains in my thoughts, and I wish him well.

"Fear does not stop death, it stops life; and worrying does not take away tomorrow's troubles, it takes away today's peace. " (Vi Keeland)

August 13, 2020

It has been just over a week since I received chemo at Dana-Farber, and I can still feel the cumulative effects of it. I am still experiencing a tingling sensation in my fingers. I still feel "foggy," the cracks on the sides of my lips have returned, and I have abdominal discomfort. The good news is that I will hopefully never have to have chemo again, and these ailments will dissipate with time.

I recently had a video conference with Dana-Farber and, for the most part, was told that I really cannot be doing any better than I am. All of my labs are pretty good. My CA19-9 was 34, and that was prior to my last chemo; it should be even lower now. My tumor measures 1.7 cm x 1.4 cm, and there is minimal vascular involvement. The only glitch that was encountered during my last CT scan was that I had a blood clot in the tip of the catheter of my port. I was told that this commonly happens. However, because of this, I was put on the blood thinner Eliquis. The plan is to remain on Eliquis for 4 - 6 weeks in order to dissolve the clot. The port will then be removed before my Whipple surgery which will be on October 1st. (As you will soon find out, the port was not removed, and I remained on Eliquis for several other months.)

I also had a video conference with my thyroid surgeon. Surgery to remove the right side of my thyroid will be in November. (It was later decided that I would complete all of my pancreatic cancer treatment before thyroid surgery.)

The surgery should take about 1 hour. I will then remain in the recovery room for around 6 hours before I am allowed to go home. I was told that even if the nodule proves to be cancerous, it does not necessarily mean that the other half of the thyroid will have to be removed.

I have begun to prep for radiation which begins next Wednesday, August 19th. The prep includes taking gas x 4 times a day as well as taking Prilosec. On Monday, I will begin to take MiraLAX. Radiation should only last one hour each day. Its side effects might include nausea and tiredness.

In general, I am doing well. I am back to my original weight of around 165. I exercise regularly and am ready to continue to do whatever has to be done to put this experience behind me.

August 19, 2020

I just completed my first round of radiation. The traffic heading into Boston was a little bit heavier than usual, but this was right around 8 a.m. I had left my house at 6:30 for an 8:30 appointment. Giving myself two hours to get to my appointment creates a less stressful venture. It allows for traffic delays, finding parking at Dana-Farber and then walking to Brigham and Women's, just a block away, where I have my treatment. I wanted to drive myself, but my friends insisted that they bring me. I feel that I have the best support system that anyone could possibly have.

They, at Brigham and Women's, were right on time as I was ushered into the treatment area at 8:30. I had to first don hospital attire, only leaving on my underwear. After passing through two metal detectors, I was brought into the treatment room. I laid down on the bed leading into the MRI. I then positioned myself as instructed and then was told to lie still. The staff adjusted my position on the bed so that I would be perfectly lined up to receive my treatment. A rigid but comfortable device, I don't know what it is called nor for what purpose it serves, was placed over my chest and abdomen. This device was then strapped to me with my arms down by my sides so that my movement was restricted. A bulb pump was placed in my left hand. If at any time I needed assistance, I was told to squeeze the bulb. Ear protection was applied, which also allowed me to listen to music of my choosing during the initial phase of the procedure. This initial phase lasted for approximately a half hour. It was during this time that all final adjustments were made in order to receive radiation. Once the radiation began, I had to use a mirror located just over my head to see a monitor behind me. On the screen, I could see an image of the inside of my body. There was also a yellow stationary circle as well as a pink one that moved with my every breath. My job was to keep the pink circle inside of the yellow. I did this by regulating my breathing and then holding my breath as long as possible once the pink circle was inside of the yellow. This process went on for about 25 minutes.

The entire process was painless, although you do have to remain perfectly still. I moved my leg for a brief moment and was immediately told not to move. There were no IVs or dye needed. I was given about 50 ml of water to drink just before the procedure. I was told to take Zofran at 8 a.m. Common side effects include nausea and tiredness. I came home and went for a bike ride.

Four more sessions left. By next Tuesday, I will be done with radiation.

The rest of my sessions went fairly smoothly. There was only one time when my procedure was delayed for about an hour. I felt bad for the person that had driven me to Boston and maintained contact with them, informing them about the delay and when I hoped I would be finished. I initially wanted to have radiation for five consecutive days but was happy that my schedule was Wednesday, Thursday, Friday, Monday, and Tuesday; it was a lot easier that way. By Friday, I was exhausted. I had been cleaning my pool for about an hour and a half. I had the vacuum inside the pool when I looked at my wife, who was outside with me and said, "I am done." I could not do any more work. I left the vacuum in the pool and went inside for a two-hour nap. When I woke, I felt better and continued cleaning the pool.

Following my last treatment, there is a gong that you hit, signifying your completion. Another battle in my war on cancer was over, at least for now.

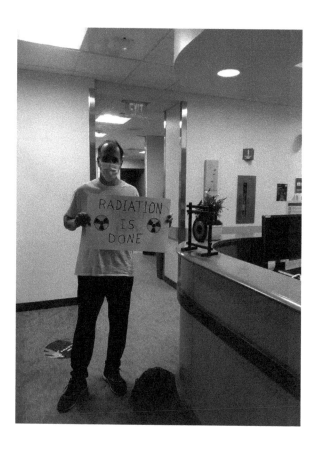

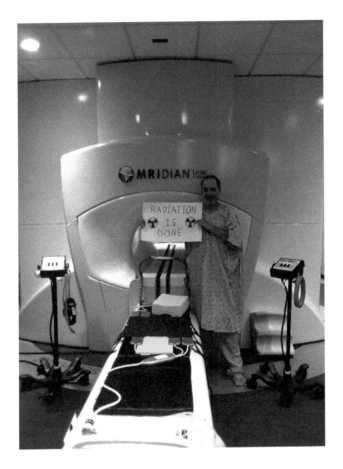

Four hundred hours of chemo and five hours of radiation have been completed. I say that these procedures are done for now, only because I do not know what the future will bring. Will I need more chemo? Will I need more radiation? I guess only time will tell.

September 9, 2020

Today I met with my Surgeon at Dana-Farber. My Whipple surgery is scheduled for October 1st. I have to be at Brigham and Women's at 5:30 a.m. Surgery is scheduled to begin at 7:30. The procedure could last anywhere from 4 - 12 hours. If possible, the Surgeon will utilize robotics to make two small incisions, rather than one larger one. This will decrease the healing time. During the Whipple surgery, the head of my pancreas, where the tumor is located, will be removed. My duodenum, as well as my gallbladder, will also be removed. A Foley catheter, as well as two drains, will be inserted and left in place for a few days. I will remain on clear liquids for a couple of days and should be up and out of bed as soon as possible. I will be in the hospital for a week. My port, which I thought was going to be taken out before surgery, will be left in place, and I am to remain on Eliquis until such time as it is removed.

Once the tumor is extracted, it will be analyzed to determine if more chemo is needed. It has been a month since my last chemo, and I still have a tingling sensation in my fingers, toes, and teeth; I hope no more chemo is warranted.

After surgery, my blood sugar will be monitored closely. It is unknown as to whether or not I will be a diabetic. One thing I have learned is that people respond to the same treatment differently. Answers to many of my questions have always been, you may or may not; it is a wait-and-see.

Yes, it continues to be a nightmare, but there are no other acceptable options, so I forge forward, continuing to do what I gotta do. So, I think it has been a month since my last chemo, a month from now, surgery will be over, and I will be back home recuperating. Two months from now, I should feel like I am feeling now as well as being cancer free. The only thing I can say is, let's do this.

Attitude is the difference between an ordeal and an adventure. (Bob Bitchin)

Today I begin what could be a four-day fasting with nothing to consume except clear liquids. I am not nervous about the Whipple surgery that I will have tomorrow. Just anxious to get it done and over. I am nervous about what the Surgeon may tell me afterward, but I am hoping for the best. I am sometimes angry that this happened to me, but I realize that I have to continue to do what must be done in regard to my treatment.

Throughout this time, I have remained active, and there is basically nothing I cannot do. I still bike regularly and have done a little running, hiking, and kayaking.

I am optimistic about a quick recovery so that I can focus on resolving my thyroid issue. I anticipate surgery to remove half of my thyroid will be in November. I am hoping that by Thanksgiving, I will be well on my way to recovery.

October 1, 2020

    I left my home with my wife at 3:30 a.m. and went to my in-law's home. My sister-in-law drove me to Brigham and Women's. I arrived earlier than necessary. Although I was told to arrive at 5:30 a.m., I did not have to arrive until 6:30. Because I had already arranged for transportation, I did not want to change my sister-in-law's schedule. She had already agreed to bring me to Boston before she had to report to work, so I did not want to impose on her with a time change. Once again, because of Covid, no one was allowed to accompany me for my surgery, so my wife waited at home to be notified of my results. The time I spent in the waiting area went by relatively quickly. There were several other people also waiting for surgery. Each one of us had an overnight bag that we had packed. The bags were collected at a counter and tagged. I felt like I was in the baggage area of an airport. When my name was called (at Dana Farber and Brigham and Women's, your first name and last initial are always announced), I followed that person into the pre-op area. I was told to get completely undressed and given a Johnny to wear. I was also given socks to put on my feet. I climbed into bed and was immediately attended to by a variety of different people. My nurse greeted me and established an IV. A tech took my blood sugar level. She was concerned about it because I believe it was over 300. She showed the reading to the doctors, but they did not appear phased. I had not eaten in several days, and just prior to going into pre-op, I had to drink a bottle of sugar water that had been given to me several days ago when I had to go to Brigham for a presurgery intake exam. I am not certain why I had to drink this, but it definitely affected my glucose level. I met with numerous different doctors that would be in the surgery room with me, two of which were anesthesiologists. Finally, after everyone had left, my surgeon arrived and asked me how I was doing. I told him that it didn't matter how I was doing. I was concerned about how he was doing. I asked him if he had a good night's sleep and if he had any type of fight with his wife or family. He laughed and said that he was fine. It seems that as soon as he left, I was being wheeled into the operating room. Again, I was greeted by many different people. I remember a mask being placed over my face. The interesting thing about this mask is that it felt more like it was made from a sort of fabric material rather than plastic. I remember being told that in a moment, I would be asked to get onto the operating table. The next thing I remember is that I was being tapped on the shoulder as my name was being called out. I said, "OK, I will get on the table now." The nurse said to me, "That was ten hours ago. You are done." I thought to myself, ten hours, where did I go? Anesthesia is amazing. I remember being worried about being placed under. Now I welcome it. It is such a great relaxing feeling. Anytime I now have any anesthesia, I offer my recovery nurse an extra $50 if she lets me sleep an extra hour. An interesting thing about surgery and going under anesthesia is that at the end of your surgical procedure, you are woken up in the operating room, you just never remember that.

I shared my hospital room with another cancer patient. I remember being wheeled into my room and asking if I was going to have to get off of my bed and onto another. Their answer was no. I said, "Good because I don't think I can do that." I don't remember much more about the rest of the evening. I don't even remember the elevator ride to my floor. I had a Foley catheter as well as two drains in my abdomen. I do remember asking to have my picture taken with the sign I had made showing that my surgery was done. I posted it on Facebook, and my son-in-law responded by saying that he was not aware that I had my wisdom teeth removed. I did not understand what he meant, and just kind of blew it off. It wasn't until the following day that I put on my reading glasses and saw the picture clearly. Wow, I was blown up like a tick. I asked why I was so swollen and was told that during my surgery, carbon dioxide was blown into my abdomen to keep it somewhat inflated. I guess that this allows for better access to the organs during the operation. Seeing how the surgery lasted ten hours, the carbon dioxide spread to all areas of my body, causing swelling everywhere. I remember tapping on my thighs, which sounded like bongos being played. One doctor said that I appeared more swollen than usual but that the carbon dioxide would eventually be absorbed by my body, and the swelling would go down. Until then, I kept on with my drum solo by beating on various areas of my body. Even after I returned home, I was still swollen for several weeks.

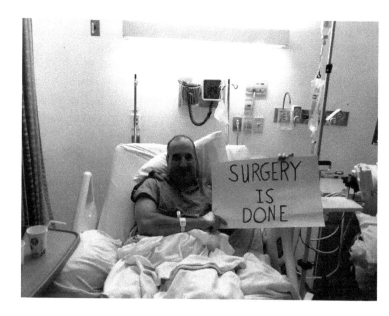

My pain was not too severe, and I was given Dilaudid for pain management as needed. I had three bags hanging from me; one was for urine from my Foley catheter, and the other two were attached to the drains leading from my abdomen. I was able to sleep fairly well that first night. Friday, was the following day. I was placed on a clear liquid diet which I tolerated quite well. I did not do much that day and tried to sleep as often as I could. I believe that on Saturday, I was given solid food. I also got out of bed and went for a short walk. On Sunday, I walked a little bit more. My nurse told me that she was going to remove my Foley catheter, and later, my drains would also be removed. It kind of felt a little strange that someone was going to do this to me. I understand that to her, it is just her job and that she probably does it all the time, but to me, it just feels different. It is not a feeling of embarrassment but more like one of passivity. People are doing things to me that I do not want them to do, and yet I don't really have much of a choice. In fact, it is the entire process; I don't want to do any of it, and yet I just put my head down, place one foot in front of the other and keep moving forward. I don't want to get back into the ring where all I do is get punched around, but I do, and I will; I will continue to do whatever it takes to defeat this demon inside of me.

I thought that the process of having my catheter removed would have been more painful than it was, but it was not too bad. It did burn the first couple of times when I peed, and my penis was left crooked. I kept looking at it, hoping that it would eventually return to normal, which it did, and so all is well that ends well. When my drains were later removed by a doctor, that was a different story. It felt like a worm was being removed from my abdomen. It was very unpleasant. I was then left with two holes in my abdomen. The drains that were used were too big for the holes to close on their own but not big enough to require several stitches. However, they did require suturing. The question was, did I want a local anesthetic injected around the site, or did I just want them stitched with no anesthetic. I was told that it would just require one suture for each incision, so I could have one needle stick and do it without anesthesia, or I could be given an injection to numb the area first and then have it sutured. I opted to go without the anesthesia and was given a piece of wood to bite down on instead – just kidding about the wood. However, the doctor ended up putting in two stitches in each incision. Yeah, it hurt a little, but whatever, it was done. Kate, my oldest daughter came by for a visit; it was nice to spend some time with her. I could only have one visitor per day and had been told that I would be going home on Monday. I welcomed the thought of going home. My mattress was not very comfortable, and my back was getting sore. My nurse wanted to know if I had a bowel movement or at least passed gas. I informed her that I had not had a bowel movement but that my roommate was now wearing a mask, and it was not because he was afraid of getting Covid.

October 5, 2020

I was discharged from the hospital today. I had initially thought that I was going to be in the hospital for at least a week, but I was discharged in only five days. I had ordered lunch and was hoping to be able to eat it before leaving, but my discharge papers, along with a wheelchair, arrived before my lunch did, and so I was quickly ushered or rather wheeled out the door to where my ride was waiting to bring me home.

Once home, I was greeted by my dog, who followed me to the couch, happy to be under a blanket and by my side. As the days passed, I began to get stronger. I had not taken any pain medication since I had left the hospital. Things appeared to be going fine until about a week later when one of my drains began to leak serosanguineous fluid.

October 14, 2020

It will be two weeks tomorrow since I had my surgery. There were 7 incisions in my abdomen, including the two drains. During this two-week period, I have spent much of my time on the couch. Each day I have gone for small walks around my neighborhood. Today I was able to walk for 2 miles, and tomorrow I will be even stronger. I have had some abdominal as well as back pain and have taken pain medication when needed. Several days ago, I had serosanguineous fluid leaking from one of my incisions. This type of leakage is common and is part of the healing process. The fluid was clear, and I did not experience any pain. It was more of a nuisance than anything else because it would leak through my dressing and get my clothes wet. Once it started to leak, I would squeeze my abdomen to get as much out as possible. I know this was probably not the thing to do, but I have a history of squeezing things – let's leave it at that. I began to cover the dressing with a face cloth, and that helped keep my clothes dry. After several days it stopped leaking.

Most of my swelling is gone, and the rice crispies sensation under my skin, due to the carbon dioxide used in surgery, is also gone in most areas; I still have some of it in my chest. I don't really have any dietary restrictions. I was advised to eat smaller, more frequent meals. My only medications are Prilosec and Eliquis.

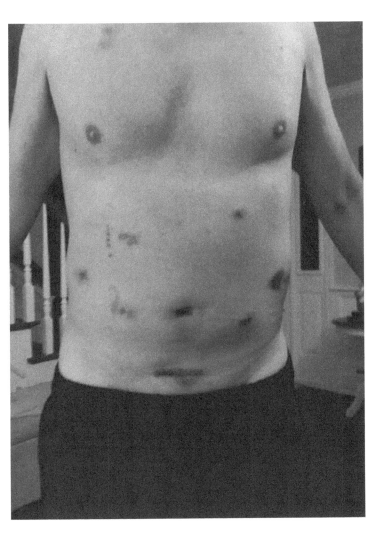

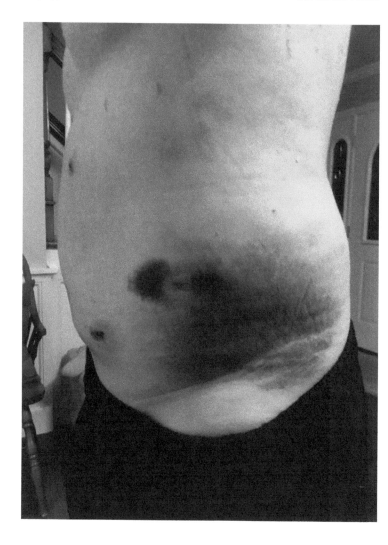

October 16, 2020

Today I met with my surgeon to discuss the results and findings of my surgery. I was very apprehensive about what was going to be said. I was hoping that I would be told that I was cancer free, but I also feared that the results would not be that good. I thought that I would come away from this meeting with either a feeling of elation or with one in which the weight of the world was on my shoulders; I came away with neither. When I was on the sidewalk outside of the Brigham, I sat for a moment and paused for reflection as to what I had just been told. I agreed with my thoughts that it was good news. My margins were clear, and they said that, as far as they were concerned, I was cancer free. Thirty-two lymph nodes had been removed, and only one had cancerous cells. Even though that lymph node was removed, I wondered how many others could have cancerous cells? I was told that I was two deviations ahead of everyone else, whatever that meant. I responded very well to both chemo and radiation; they did what they were supposed to do. One incision site is infected. I will be placed on antibiotics, maybe Bactrim. Whether or not I receive more chemo will depend on what the oncologist says; I should find out today. My surgeon is not opposed to me having more chemo, just as a precaution. An appointment will be made for thyroid surgery and removal of the port. I should have more information as soon as I hear from my oncologist. The surgeon seemed to be leaning towards more chemo just to be certain to kill any other cells not found. The tingling sensation in my hands and feet could be permanent, and I was told I would be on Prilosec for life to prevent any ulcerations at the anastomoses sites. My results left me feeling neither excited nor depressed, more like in a limbo state.

An anastomosis is a connection between two things. During my Whipple procedure, the head of my pancreas, where my tumor was located, was removed, as was my gallbladder and duodenum. My stomach was also separated from my intestine. Then, my pancreas and stomach were reattached to another part of my intestine. The places where they were reattached are known as anastomoses. Prilosec is used to prevent damage at those sites by neutralizing stomach acids. Normally people take Prilosec for acid reflux and heartburn; I do not have those conditions.

October 28, 2020

Today I met with my oncologist, and it was mutually agreed upon that I will have another four rounds of chemo. He is not sure if the chemo will help, but he said if we want to be as aggressive as possible, then we should do another four rounds. I agreed with him, and so I will begin chemo in two weeks. He initially said that it was my choice to make and that I could take a week if I wanted to decide. I told him that I would do whatever he suggested. Next week I will go for a CT scan to be used as a new baseline. My port will stay in, and I will remain on Eliquis. I will not have thyroid surgery until chemo is done.

Mentally I am OK with this decision, and physically I feel strong enough to continue the fight. I have already come this far; I can do another four rounds just to be on the "safe side." I still have a lot of things to do in my life. I would hate for cancer to return and would always wonder that it might not have if I had done another four rounds of chemo.

November 9, 2020

On Wednesday, I begin my second series of chemotherapy. I am scheduled for 4 more rounds, which will be a lot better than the initial 8. I am recovering quite well from my surgery. Although I still have abdominal discomfort, the same as which I had prior to surgery, I have no pain related to the surgery itself.

I would like to thank everyone again for all your support. Specifically, I would like to thank you for the nearly 100-car parade that passed by my house; I was truly surprised. The financial support. The countless prayers and well wishes. The numerous cards that continue to come in, often more than one from the same people. The flowers. The puzzle, which I finished even though my wife said I cheated. The masses said, and candles lit. The statues of angles. The chakra stones, which I always bring with me to chemo. The walks on the beach, the woods, and in the Blue Hills. The kayak adventure. The cutting of my lawn and taking out of my trash. The stethoscope; I am still not working Christmas Day. The Kindle Fire; I'll figure it out. The books. The socks and shirts. The "You Got This" saying, which I look at every day. The suggestions of what to watch on TV. The food (now don't be jealous) but it has included: a clam boil, lobster, steak, fish chowder, stuffed quahogs, fish, crepes, meat pies, linguica rolls, spinach rolls, pasta, shepherd's pie, stuffed peppers, homemade loaves of bread, soups like kale, chicken, vegetable, beef, various lunch sandwiches, roast beef and meatball subs, Hawaiian pizza, Portuguese rolls, hummus, and other Lebanese foods I can't pronounce or spell, banana nut bread, brownies, cookies, sweet rice, ice cream. Are you full yet? If I forgot something, it's because I ate it too quickly; send more so I can remember. Also, thank you for the weekly grocery shopping and all the rides back and forth to Boston. Finally, I would like to thank you for the hours I have spent talking with you on the phone as well as texting; I truly appreciate all the advice you have given me, as well as the foolish discourse we shared. Lastly, I would like to thank my wife again for her 24/7 support. I know it has been difficult for her as well.

ROUND NINE (11/11/20)

Today I met with my NP. I thought it was going to be with my doctor, but meeting with my NP is fine. Prior to meeting with her, I had blood work. We were all pleased with the results.   Even though all of my values were still not within normal limits, most were. In particular, my CA19-9, a cancer marker, was 9. The normal range for anyone, including someone without cancer, is 0 - 34. The highest level that I remember talking about was 135, although I may have seen a report saying it was 178. I also have a liver enzyme, I believe ALP, that remains elevated at 171. I believe the normal high is around 134, but I am not sure, I just know that it hasn't changed since May, and they don't seem concerned about it. I was told that because of all the chemo I have had, it might take a while for my liver enzymes to return to normal. My white blood cell count is now within normal limits, and although chemo is going to decrease it, the Neulasta I will be taking on Friday after I come off the pump is going to elevate it above normal.

We talked about my Whipple surgery and how I had only one lymph node out of 32 that was removed during surgery, which contained cancerous cells. I thought that was good, but she did not appear very impressed and said that it was a normal finding. What she was very excited about was that all of the margins surrounding my tumor were clear. She was also concerned with the neuropathy I am experiencing in the tips of my fingers and soles of my feet. She was most concerned about my feet. My fingertips feel still tingly, and my feet, when I walk barefoot, feel as though there is about a half inch of extra padding under them. She said that some people actually have a hard time walking and that this condition could be permanent. It is caused by Oxaliplatin, one of the chemo meds, and so she is going to reduce it by one and see how I do. I did not experience these effects until after around the fifth chemo treatment. It was only then that they would not go away. It was also then that I began to experience hair loss, but only on the top of my head, and it has all grown back.

I think feel that the session went well. I felt almost as if I could have driven myself home, although I am deeply grateful that I did not have to, and for the first time, I did not have to stop and pee.

When I got home, I put on the movie Jaws and took a 2-hour nap. Don't ask me why, but when I want to nap, I turn on Jaws. I can't even tell you how many times I have slept through that movie. I woke up feeling slightly nauseated, and by the time I walked upstairs to my bedroom, I was more nauseated, diaphoretic, and pale. I took Compazine for nausea and Xanax to help me sleep. I cannot take Zofran until my pump comes out on Friday. In general, I feel okay. One of the problems that I am having is that when I pass gas, I stink; I mean, I can't even stand it. I know it's not a pleasant thing to talk about, but I am just trying to let you know what happens. Also, I believe my breath has a strange odor because my dog is "hitting-on" my mouth again before she crawls under the bed covers; yes, she sleeps with me. An interesting thing is that for months prior to my cancer diagnosis, she "hit" on my breath. Maybe it was something that should be paid attention to, although your doctor might think you're somewhat nuts when you tell him/her the reason for your visit is that your dog is smelling your breath.

November 20, 2020

Today marks a full week off of chemo. Here is a recap of my chemo process. Every other Wednesday, I go to Dana-Farber for treatment. Because of Covid, no visitors are allowed, so my family remains at home waiting for my return 10 hours later. It takes exactly 3.5 hours to receive all of the chemo given to me at Dana-Farber, but there is blood work, a doctor's visit, and the chemo has to be prepared. Then I receive another 46 hours of chemo, at home, via a pump that is attached to me through the port in my chest. On Friday, the pump is removed, and recovery begins.

What It Is Like for Me

Wednesday - Chemo Day

After a couple of hours of receiving chemo, I have to pee every 15 - 20 minutes. My head begins to get a little foggy. The thought of food makes me nauseated. I am happy when I am finished and leave without difficulty. My ride is waiting for me outside. Once home, I have something to eat and try to take a nap on the couch. When I awake, I take Compazine for nausea and Xanax to help me sleep. I then go to bed.

Thursday and Friday

I remain on the couch and in my PJs. Friday, after the pump is removed, I shower, get dressed, and go outside to get some fresh air. I feel pretty good; not too much head fog.

Saturday

The fog sets in, and I am tired and spend most of the day on the couch.

Sunday

Fatigued - much worse than being tired. No energy to do anything. Another day on the couch.

Monday and Tuesday (finally have a bowel movement)

Begin to exercise; bike, walk, etc.

Wednesday until the following Tuesday

The fog lifts a little more each day, and I increase my activities.

The following day is chemo, and the process begins again. I know what to expect, and so I will just play it out as described above. My last round at Dana-Farber will be December 23rd, with the pump coming off on Christmas Day.

I have been lucky in that I have never really been sick with any of my treatments. I have neuropathy in my hands and feet. The corners of my mouth are cracked again. I have increased saliva and post-nasal drip. I am having a hard time maintaining my weight. If I lose any of my hair, it may occur next month, but it should grow back.

It's not easy, but it's gotta get done cause I got stuff to do later.

You may not be able to control every situation and its outcome, but you can control your attitude and how you deal with it. (Adrianna Serrato)

ROUND TEN (11/25/20)

GETTING IT DONE

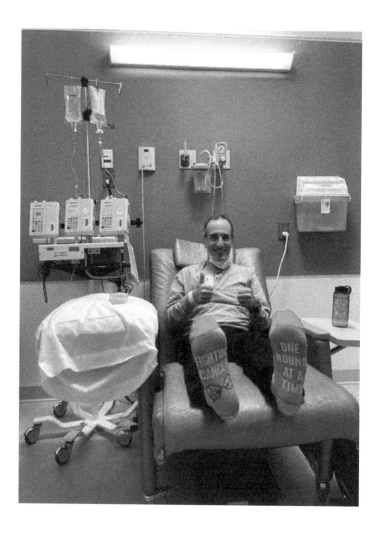

Every other week for about 6 months, I would spend 3.5 hours, basically in this position, with chemo and other medications being infused into my body.

I cannot thank Dana-Farber enough for all they have done for me. I would not be alive today if it were not for them. You never know when your life will completely change. A year ago, I never thought I would have been diagnosed with pancreatic cancer. I am hoping today, thanks to Dana-Farber, that I am cancer free. Again, thanks to everyone at Dana-Farber for all they do, and thanks to everyone out there for your continued support.

Molly is my NP; she is awesome. I will meet with her tomorrow just prior to my second to last chemo treatment. She invited me to her retirement party, which is probably 30+ years away, I plan to be there. OK, so actually, I invited myself but whatever.

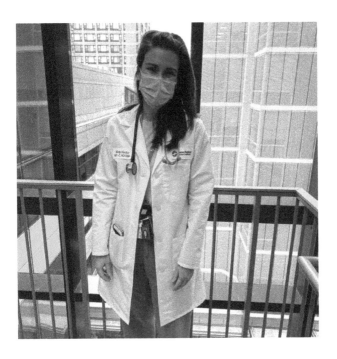

ROUND ELEVEN (12/9/20)

One more round to go. I know that I have said this before, but hopefully, this time, I will be right. Throughout this entire process, I have tried to listen to my body and have been aware of how I feel and the changes that I have gone through. I hope that I caught this disease before it spread to other parts of my body. It is important that you pay attention to what your body is telling you and act accordingly. Seek medical attention sooner than later if you suspect something is not right.

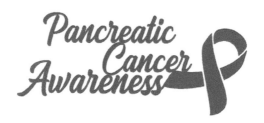

December 18, 2020

Yesterday I spent the day moving snow at my house, my mom's, daughter's, mother-in-law's, and aunt's. I have a utility trailer which I use to transport a snowblower. When I returned home, it was getting dark. I backed the trailer into my driveway. When I woke up this morning and looked out my window, this image was made by my tire tracks.

I am really not superstitious, but sometimes I find myself looking for signs - signs for what? I am not really sure. Maybe in the hope that things will be alright or perhaps for direction regarding future decisions. Seeing these two heart-like images left me with the message that everything would be alright, that I would be alright. I also remember at one point, crows seemed to be following me around as I walked around my neighborhood. It is said that seeing a crow means that someone from the spiritual world is trying to communicate with you. I don't recall how many crows I kept seeing, for I know that different numbers may indicate different things, but I again tried to imagine that it was a positive sign.

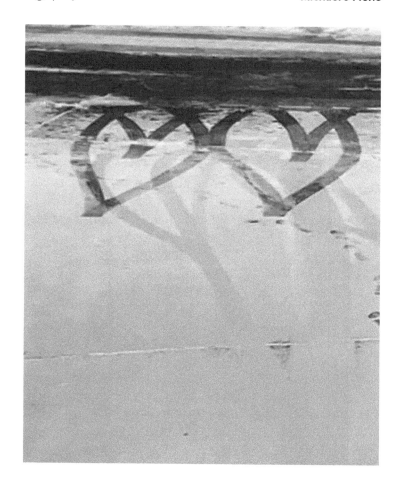

ROUND TWELVE (12/23/20)

I am now in my twelfth round of chemo. Once I complete this round on Friday, I will have received nearly 600 hours of chemo. In addition to that, I have had more than 2 hours of radiation and a 10-hour Whipple surgery.

- My doctor seemed pleased with my progress. Here are a few updates.

- Remain on Eliquis as long as I have port

- The greatest chance for cancer to return is within the first year

- No Covid or flu vaccine for about a month. Vaccine not as effective while on or recently receiving chemo

- Return to Dana-Farber every three months for the next five years

Perhaps the best news that I received from my doctor occurred just prior to me walking out of the room when he told me that my port would be coming out soon. I remember him initially saying that my port would be left in place for about a year following all treatment. To me, this news meant that I was doing extremely well. I can't even begin to tell you the joy I felt walking out of this meeting.

December 25, 2020

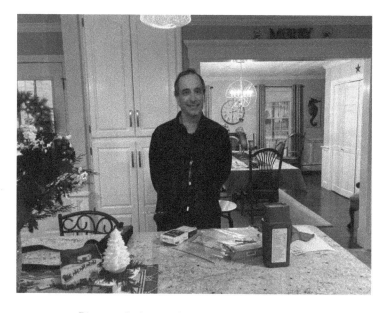

Pictured above, I am receiving my last
chemo treatment – hopefully, this time for good.
MERRY CHRISTMAS TO MYSELF

January 1, 2021

HAPPY NEW YEAR

A year ago, no one had any idea what 2020 would bring. We all shared loss: The death of a family member or friend, missed vacations, loss of a job, financial instability, canceled events, and on and on. Yet we rejoiced in the birth of a child, a marriage or engagement, the addition of a new family member, pet or friend, a new job, house or car, and on and on.

A year ago, I had no idea that I had cancer. I had no idea what I would have to endure for most of 2020. I have a port in my chest, my gallbladder has been removed, as well as the head of my pancreas, a portion of my stomach, and my duodenum. These account for some of my 2020 losses. What I gained in return is an entire village of people that have supported me in my battle against cancer. I have become closer to my family and friends. I have rekindled old relationships and realized how important we all are to each other.

I wish that I did not have to go through all that I did, but it was my fate, my destiny, and now a part of my history. I cannot erase 2020, and maybe I don't want to. It is said that if a group of people enter into a room and remove their "cross," which represents all of their life burdens, share those burdens with everyone else, and then in the end, could choose any cross to leave with, the majority of people would choose their own.

There are no certainties in life besides nature's plan, so live for today, for yesterday is gone forever, and tomorrow may never come.

January 14, 2021

Today I returned to Dana-Farber for blood work and a CT scan of my chest, abdomen, and pelvis. Within 5 minutes of having my blood drawn, I had some of my results. Within 45 minutes before my CT scan, I had all of my results. By Friday morning, I had the results of the CT scan of my chest. The report indicated that the scan of my abdomen and pelvis would come in a separate report. Every other time I had a CT scan, I received the results of my chest, abdomen, and pelvis at the same time, read by the same radiologist. This time it was different. By Friday afternoon, I still had no results for my abdomen and pelvis, so I called Dana-Farber. I was told that the results would be sent to me within 24 hours. The weekend came and went with still no results. I can't even tell you the number of times I checked the portal for them. On Tuesday, I called again. I said that I had an appointment with my urologist that afternoon and wanted to show him the results. I was told that the results would be sent to me shortly, but they never came. Later I learned that no one ever read the scans. I kind of feel that someone "dropped the ball" in not reading the scans, which caused me a great deal of distress. I think we have to realize that what we do or say can impact someone's life. If only that radiologist had read all of my scans, as every other radiologist had done before, I would not have had to experience all the anxiety I did. Whatever it is that you do, please do it honestly and to the best of your ability. It really doesn't hurt to "go out of your way" for someone else, even just a little. It can have a great impact on their life.

This morning I received my results, and this afternoon I had a virtual conference with my oncologist. Let me begin by saying that most of the results of my blood work fell within normal limits. My CT scans looked pretty good as well. My oncologist was very pleased with all of my results and said that, at this point, I no longer have any signs of cancer. The plan right now is to have my port removed next month and to come off of Eliquis in March. I will have more blood work in three months, and another CT scan in six. I can't even tell you how happy I am as tears of joy roll down my face. It has been a long hard road. I know that there is always a chance of cancer returning, but right now, I have to believe that I am CANCER-FREE.

On Tuesday, January 26th, I will have the right side of my thyroid removed. Just one more hurdle that I will overcome.

Again, I can't thank all of you enough for all of your support. I also cannot fully express all of my gratitude to all the faculty and staff at Dana-Farber Cancer Institute/ Brigham and Women's Hospital, in particular my oncologist, surgeon, and their entire team. Without them, I would not be here today.

January 25, 2021

As stated before, my cancer treatments have ended, hopefully forever. The next time I have to have blood work will be in April. One of the main things that will be looked at is "cancer markers." In my case, that is CA 19-9, as well as CEA. Cancer antigen 19-9 (CA 19-9) is a protein that exists on the surface of certain cancer cells. It can be found, in small amounts, even in the blood of healthy people. At high levels, it is often a sign of pancreatic cancer, but it can indicate other types of cancer, as well as noncancerous disorders such as gallstones, pancreatitis, bile duct blockage, liver disease, and even cystic fibrosis.

Carcinoembryonic antigen (CEA), another cancer marker, is also usually present, at low levels, in the blood of healthy individuals. Certain types of cancer can cause this level to rise as well. The normal range is between 0 - 3.7 mg/ml. I have always remained within the normal range.

Every three months for the next five years, I will anxiously await the results of these two cancer numbers. Hopefully, they will always fall within normal limits.

Tomorrow I will undergo surgery to remove the right side of my thyroid. As of right now, I still don't know what time my surgery will be. Initially, I was told that it would be at 7:30 a.m. I have to be at Brigham and Women's two hours early, so I scheduled someone to pick me up from my house at 4 a.m. Then I was told to call today between

2 - 4 to find out the time. Oh well, I will just bring a book. I have nothing else to do anyway. It is only one more hurdle in life to overcome. I was told the surgery would take about one hour. I will spend six hours in recovery, and then I will come home - no big deal. Again, you just do what you gotta do.

January 26, 2021

Today I had the right side of my thyroid removed in a procedure called a thyroid lobectomy, also known as a partial thyroidectomy or hemithyroidectomy. I arrived at Brigham and Women's early and first thing in the morning. The receptionist was far from friendly, as all of the others had been. There were numerous people in the waiting area, and I found a seat at the back of the room. I was not there long when someone came into the room and called out my first name only. This was completely different than at any other time. All other times, the patient's first name and last initial are called. Obviously, I was not the only Michael in the room, and another person got up and went over to the woman. He asked the woman for the last name of the person she was looking for, and her response to him, in a sarcastic tone, was, "Is there more than one Michael here?' He replied that there was, and so when she called out the last name, it happened to be mine.

I followed her into the pre-op room and was told to undress and put on a johnny with the open end at the back. I could leave on my socks. I did so immediately and climbed into bed, and coved myself up with a sheet and blanket. A short time later, I decided that I should go to the bathroom. As I was walking around pre-op, I realized that my back end was probably exposed. I thought to myself, I have already been through so much. I don't even care. I feel that my dignity was lost a long time ago. Returning from the bathroom, I climbed back into bed. I nurse came over to me, but only for a brief moment, and then she left. I was there alone for a longer period than I had ever been. The patient next to me had a nurse that was very attentive to her, but mine seemed aloof. I could tell from the activity going on behind the closed curtain next to me that this patient was extremely anxious about her procedure. When her nurse passed by my bed, she looked at me and said that I looked very relaxed. I thought to myself, with all that I have gone through already, this was nothing.

Finally, a person arrived at my bedside and introduced herself as the resident anesthesiologist, and said that she was going to start my IV. I thought, great, who better to start my IV. She easily found a vein in my hand (my veins stick out of my hands and arms and are readily accessible) and, using a small needle, injected my hand with lidocaine or some other local anesthetic. She did this so that I could not feel her starting the IV. She applied the tourniquet and attempted to insert a needle. Although she hit the vein, she failed to start the IV. I thought to myself, how could she have blown that vein. As I paramedic, I start IV's all the time and would consider myself an easy "stick." I can't even remember when someone else failed to insert an IV in my hand or arm on the first attempt. Because I am on Eliquis, I began to bleed through the injection site. I could not believe that this had happened. I was very relaxed before, but now I started to feel slightly anxious. As she was cleaning up the blood, now over a part of my hand, a male in a white lab coat approached my bed. His ID indicated that he was a doctor. He asked me how I was and said, "So we are going to be removing the left side of your thyroid today." I looked at him and said, "No, it is the right side." He looked at me and said, "Are you sure?" I could not believe what I was hearing. First, the anesthesiologist missed my IV, and now this guy wants to remove the wrong side of my thyroid. I was now sweating, and yes, I was now quite anxious. After

I brief moment, he came back and said, "You are correct. It is the right side." I thought to myself, yeah, no kidding. My hand was now cleaned up, and the anesthesiologist was about to make a second attempt. She once again went to inject the IV site with lidocaine, and I told her, "Please don't do that. Just start the IV." She looked at me and said, "Boy, you are brave." I thought, the IV did not really hurt anyway; it hurts just as much as the small needle you are using to inject the local anesthetic. Why get stuck twice when once will work. The second time was a charm, and she started the IV without incident. As she was finishing up, other people began to come to my bedside to discuss my procedure with me. I made certain to tell each one of them that it was the right side of my thyroid and not the left. Finally, my surgeon arrived, and I made sure to tell him the same. He kind of smiled and said, "Yes, I know." Perhaps he had heard about what happened with the other doctor. I asked him if he was going to mark the site with a marker, and he said that he was and then proceeded to do so. The anesthesiologist then wheeled me into the operating room, nearly striking another person in the process. At last, I was in the operating room. I was placed next to the operating table and told to get on it myself, so I shimmied over from my bed onto the table. Once I was settled, a mask was placed over my face, and I was told to think happy thoughts. I could feel myself going out. It is actually kind of a pleasant feeling; I was relaxed at this point, and I did not attempt to fight it.

When I woke up, I was in the recovery room. I felt how one is expected to feel following surgery. I was a bit groggy and felt only slight discomfort in my neck. At one point, I had to pee, and so I informed my nurse, who then came to me with a urinal, and told me not to get out of bed. She closed the curtain, and in good male fashion, I immediately go out of bed and stood up to pee. Without me knowing, she opened the curtain, saw me standing there, and gave me hell for doing so. I was in the recovery room for perhaps a few hours before I was discharged. I was wheeled out to meet my wife and Diane, my son-in-law's mother, who would be driving me home. It had just begun to snow, and we were expecting about 8 inches of the white stuff. The drive home was easy but slow going due to the road conditions. When I arrived home, I rested as I normally do after surgery. However, the following day, I felt well enough to move snow using a snowblower and shovel and did so for about 5 hours. I had no pain and only minimal discomfort. The surgical incision left me with only a small scar on the fold of my neck, hardly visible. I do not have to take any thyroid medication; the other half of my thyroid is producing enough hormones to maintain my health. The pathology report indicated that the mass was a follicular adenoma - a benign, non-cancerous, encapsulated tumor.

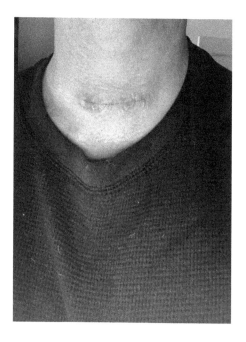

March 10, 2021

One week from today, I am scheduled to have my port removed. It has been nearly a year since it was implanted in my chest, and my journey began. I am doing OK and have regained my strength. My biggest issue remains with not being able to gain weight. I am maintaining my weight, and I am comfortable with it, but for the amount I eat, I should weigh as much as a hippopotamus. Anyway, a month after the port is removed, I can stop taking the blood thinner Eliquis. At that point, the only meds I will be on are Prilosec and Creon. My blood sugars are fine, as well as my thyroid levels. On April 19th, I will return to Dana-Farber for labs. Hopefully, my CA 19-9 will be within normal limits.

March 12, 2021

OK, so I know you are not going to believe this, but... I was at my mom's house earlier this afternoon. I wanted to cut some branches from a tree that were near and against wires. I was up in the tree about 9 feet when I slipped and fell. I thought I was OK until I saw my deformed left wrist. My mom's neighbor drove me to St. Luke's in New Bedford, Massachusetts. I have to say that they were fantastic. They did a great job of taking care of me. I ended up breaking my lower left arm, both my radius, and ulna, along with my right thumb. The good news is that the CT scan did not reveal any masses in my pancreas. They reduced the fracture by lining up the bone ends and putting on a cast. At this point, no surgery is needed. I will have to see an orthopedic surgeon for a follow-up visit. I guess this is the end of my tree climbing. They are going to love me at Dana-Farber when I let them know. Anyway, the journey continues only now down a different path. A purple ribbon is symbolic of pancreatic cancer, hence the purple cast.

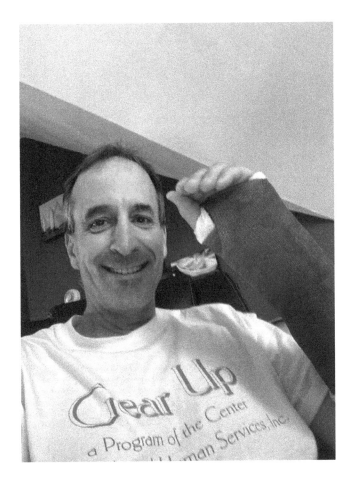

Life is a journey meant to be lived, and as we age, our faces and our body show signs of our struggle and the adversity we have overcome. Embrace your triumphs as well as your defeats for the marks they have left, visible or not, are all part of your journey and help define who you are.

March 17, 2021

Almost a year ago, my cancer journey began with the surgical implantation of a power port on the right side of my chest. Today that port was removed. Lying in bed next to me (wait, we were not in the same bed. He was on his own on the other side of a curtain, glad I got that out) was a gentleman just beginning his journey, as his port was being implanted in his chest wall. I remember being in his position and seeing another gentleman having his port removed just as I was about to. I remember how anxious I felt when I began this journey. It has been a long year, and the struggles have been hard and painful, but I am still here, grateful for each day.

April 9, 2021

I was diagnosed with pancreatic cancer a year ago today;

It is difficult to believe that my life would turn out this way.

Six months of chemo and radiation too,

You can't even imagine what I have been through.

Five surgeries have left my body scarred;

My journey has been trying, arduous, and hard.

But I have not ventured alone;

For you have been with me, and together we have grown.

I thank you for everything you have done for me this year;

You have taught me that faith, hope, and love are stronger than fear.

There is so much more for me to do and so much more to say,

But for now, I think back on how far I have come since Diagnosis Day.

April 12, 2021

Today I went to Dana-Farber for labs. My appointment was for 10:30. I left my house just before 8:30 so that I would have plenty of time to get there. I set my cruise control to 65 and enjoyed the ride. I encountered a little bit of construction on 495, but it wasn't too bad. I traveled around the Blue Hills in Milton (which, by the way, is a great place to hike) through Mattapan and took 203 and the Jamaica Plain into Boston. The total distance is around 60 miles, and it took me an hour and a half to get there. Due to Covid, parking is free in the Dana-Farber garage, and you do not have to get your ticket validated. It took 13 minutes, from the time I exited my car until the time I returned, which included checking in on the first and second floors, a brief bathroom stop, and blood work.

I was a little disappointed to see that my alkaline phosphatase, an enzyme found in the liver, was still elevated. The normal high is 129; mine is 213. The last time I had it checked, it was 205. I wouldn't have minded if it was still elevated but had come down and not gone up. My MCH, which checks for the average amount of hemoglobin, was also slightly elevated but had come down since the last time. All of my other lab values were within normal limits. Most importantly, my CA19-9, or cancer marker, was 7. This is the lowest it has ever been.

April 14, 2021

Today I had a virtual conference with my nurse practitioner oncologist. She said that all of my results were great. She is not certain why my alkaline phosphatase is still elevated, most likely still due to all the chemo, but she will continue to monitor it. She again stated that I would have to be on Prilosec for life to protect the anastomoses done during surgery.

October 1, 2021

Today is my Whippleversary. It was one year ago when I underwent a 10-hour surgery to remove a cancerous tumor from the head of my pancreas. Besides Prilosec, the only other med that I take, as needed, is Creon, a pancreatic enzyme that helps with the absorption of nutrients. I weigh 158, and no matter what or how much I eat, I don't gain weight. I know that for many of you, this just breaks your heart, and you get all teared up, but for me, it is a constant reminder that things aren't working the way they used to. Also, and I know that this too is going to break your heart, my cholesterol is the lowest it has been in years, and my blood sugars are normal.

Mornings are spent in the bathroom. If I have to be somewhere, I have to plan on getting up a little earlier to account for this time. I still have some abdominal discomfort from time to time, but in general, I would say I feel ok. I will return to Dana Farber on October 20th for blood work and to meet with my nurse practitioner. Just a few weeks ago, I did not realize my appointment was on that date. I knew that it was in October, just like I realized that sometime in January, I again returned for labs and a CT scan, but I did not really think about it; now, it is the one thing that plagues my mind. On October 20th, I will leave my house at 6 AM. My labs are at 8, and my appointment with my NP is at 9. As you can infer, I am already experiencing some anxiety as the day approaches. After obtaining the results of my labs, I will either feel as though I am floating or carrying the weight of my car as I drive home. Hopefully, it is the former that I will feel, but should it be the latter, I am ready to continue the fight. I think the worst part about that whole day is that I now have to pay for parking. During the entire time of my treatment, parking, due to Covid, was free. Cancer sucks.

Because my surgery was performed robotically, there is minimal scarring. Others that have had this same procedure have been left with large scars across their entire abdomen. Some of my scars resemble gunshot wounds. I also have a scar inside of my umbilicus.

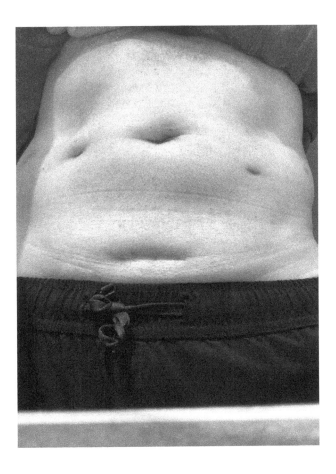

IN CONCLUSION

There is a commercial on television about St Jude's Hospital and children with cancer. Several pediatric patients give a brief statement. One such statement is from a young girl who says, "The hardest thing about cancer is knowing that you have it." Looking at her, there is a calmness and resolve in her eyes. It is the same feeling and expression that I share. It is a horrible feeling knowing that you have cancer. You really can't believe that this is now a part of your life. You wish that you could just delete it, fall asleep, and when you wake up, realize that it was only a bad dream, but it is not. It is reality. It is my reality. I hope that my journey provided you with some insight as to what it is like to have to face and deal with such a terrible illness. As I have said before, this is my journey, and although it may be reflective of what one might go through, it is by far not completely inclusive of what others experience. Hopefully, someday, we will live in a world devoid of cancer, but until that time, never ever give up hope. Stay safe.

ACKNOWLEDGEMENTS

In many stories, once readers get to the acknowledgment section, they continue no further. I encourage you to continue to read for these people, and the roles they played in my journey helped in my treatment process. Without them, my journey would have been a lot more arduous. I cannot thank them enough.

When faced with trying times, many people shut down; they retreat and keep things to themselves. I prefer to open up and discuss my feelings, to allow others into my life. No person is an island unto themselves. We rely on each other. No person knows more than we all collectively do. I believe that people inherently want to help others in times of need and so why not let them. If you let people into your life, you will find that you will have an entire village to rely on, an army to help you get through trying times. Let these people in; let them help, and find comfort in the fact that you are not in this fight alone.

My journey kind of started with a large parade of supporters that passed by my home. I would like to thank the Mattapoisett Police Department for leading the charge and directing traffic.

New Bedford Emergency Medical Services for their financial support. Thank you to all the EMTs and Paramedics for your donation.

The Rochester Fire Department for their financial support. Thank you to all the EMTs and Paramedics for your donation. Thank you for the clambake dinner; I was so excited when you arrived at my house with enough food for several days.

Cindy Dawicki and Melissa O'Dowd for being neighborly and bringing over food.

Michelle Carrier-Trail, for all the cards and words of advice and inspiration.

Bill Heydt, Seannine Tveit, Carol Ventura, Rick Huston, and Pat Gifford for the pizza party out on the deck.

Peter Letendre and Christie Moore-Letendre for all the flowers and cards.

Bev Tavares for the homemade kale soup, and her husband Gary Tavares, for checking in on me after I had eaten it, to make sure that I did not get sick or die.

Pat Costa for the left-over pasta; it was the first thing I ate one day when returning from chemo.

Wally Norcross, for all the text messages checking in on my well-being and for all the laughs.

Sarah O'Conner for the chakra stones, which I brought with me to every chemo session.

Ann Collins, for all your support and for sharing your cancer journey with me. (*May you rest in peace*)

Carin Walker Courtney, one of my former 8th-grade students now living in Texas, for the generous gift card to a local pizza restaurant. At some point during my chemo, I had a craving for red meat. I can't even tell you how many roast beef subs I was able to purchase using your card. Thank you.

Karen LaFlamme for the haircut out on the back deck as well as the fresh fish, which was used to make a fantastic meal.

Lisa Devlin for the lobster dinner. The shell was so hard I needed pliers to crack it, but it was very delicious. I took my time eating, and it took almost an hour to finish, but I savored every bite. I had never enjoyed a meal so much. My thoughts at the time were, maybe this is the way all meals should be eaten; by taking one's time and enjoying the moment. I guess the same philosophy could be applied to many other life events.

Diane and Andy Setera for all the different types of food items.

Jeanne Motyl for all the food and the puzzle. I am really not a puzzle person, but I truly enjoyed making this one. It kept me occupied for quite a while.

Rick and Amy Huston not only brought food to my house but had it delivered as well; that was a real surprise and a great idea. Thanks for the cancer socks as well.

Rose David for all the food every single week.

Jeanne Duggan for all the banana nut bread following every chemo session.

Dan Lebelle for cutting my grass

Danny Parker for cutting my grass, taking in the trash, and just keeping an eye on things around my house. It was a comfort knowing that I could rely on you to watch over my property.

Pat Gifford and John Vessella for the countless hours of text messaging. There were many times when I did not feel like watching TV or doing anything else. You kept me so busy and entertained that time passed a lot quicker than it would have if I had nothing to do. You played a huge role throughout my entire journey. You constantly checked in on me, and sometimes we would text for hours, just about stupid shit. John, thanks for all the phone conversations as well.

A big thank you to the following for all of the rides – this journey would not have been possible without you.

Wayne Robin, Joe Callanan, Paul Sardinha (Thanks, Paul, for all the spinach and linguica rolls), Jim Mahaney, Carol Mahaney, Dave Morey, Rick Huston, Jamie Benoit (also for all the food and the "Grandma's Turkey Dinner Sandwich which you brought for me during the ride home from Dana Farber). Patty Keefe and Pam Duphily, who tag-teamed with each other. (Patty, along with Pam, would pick me up at Dana Farber and then drive me to a park-in-ride near Patty's home. I would then get into Pam's car, and she would drive me the rest of the way home.) Bob Jeffrey and Diane Lash, who I could always rely on for a ride anytime I needed one. Thank you, Diane, for all of the food you would often bring to my house and for the Kindle Fire. Betty Duggan, who I think brought me to every surgical procedure I had. Robert (Bobby) Medeiros for all the rides, walks, and Hawaiian pizza.

Jim Duggan, along with Betty Duggan, for the weekly grocery shopping.

My basenji Bella, who literally never left my side. I believe she actually enjoyed all the time we spent together.

My daughters Kate Lash and Mikayla Chouinard, along with their husbands David Lash and Dan Chouinard, for their everlasting love and support.

My wife Ann for going through this journey with me and protecting me from getting sick during the Covid pandemic, cleaning every single item that was brought into our home. I know that it was difficult for her as well.

To all those that supported me in some way, sending cards and following me on Facebook, I truly appreciate everything that you have done.

I must also recognize my medical team. If not for them, you would not be reading this now.

David Clark, DO, my primary care physician, ordered the tests necessary to find my tumor.

Paul Sepe, MD, my gastroenterologist, took a biopsy of my tumor and placed a stent in my bile duct, clearing up my jaundice.

Ellen Marqusee, MD, my endocrinologist, took a biopsy of my thyroid.

Matthew Nehs, MD, my general surgeon, removed half of my thyroid.

Thomas Clancy, MD, who performed my Whipple surgery, I have no idea how you can operate and stay focused for such a long period of time.

Taylor Murphy RN, my oncology nurse who gave me all of my chemos, counseled me for an hour prior to my first treatment, provided me with IT support, brought me snacks, and cared for my wellbeing; we know who does all the work around the hospital.

Molly Nestor, NP, my oncology nurse practitioner, with whom I meet every six months. I will be at your retirement party.

Brian Wolpin, MD, my primary oncologist. You give life and provide hope to so many. Thank you so much.

To all of the staff and faculty at Dana Farber Cancer Institute and Brigham and Women's Hospital, your support, professionalism, and kindness are truly appreciated; you have saved the lives of so many. THANK YOU!

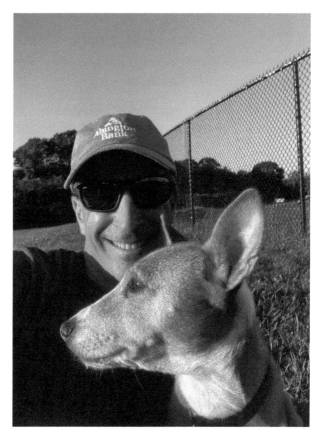

Bella and me at Fort Taber in the south end
of New Bedford.

Printed in the USA
CPSIA information can be obtained
at www.ICGtesting.com
LVHW051658270823
756436LV00011B/581

9 781916 770096